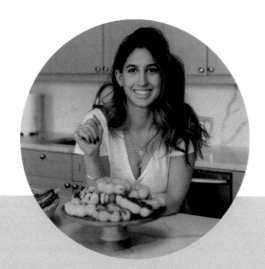

Protein Snack Queen High-Protein Cookbook

100 QUICK, SHORTCUT, HIGH-PROTEIN, LOWER-CALORIE MEALS & SNACKS

BY ASHLEY POLADIAN

THE PROTEIN SNACK QUEEN

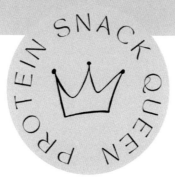

Hey There!
I'm Ashley!

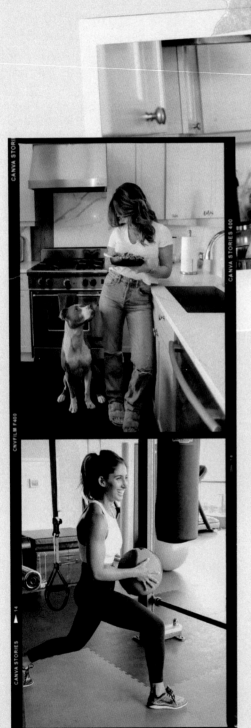

Thank you so much for purchasing my first-ever COOKBOOK! As an evidence-based Fitness and Nutrition Coach, I specialize in helping my clients lose body fat and build muscle using convenient, approachable, and sustainable methods. The truth is, I am NOT a chef – I'm more like a 'food assembler' with a keen understanding of how foods play a role in the fat loss and muscle development process. I shy away from elaborate recipes for two reasons: 1. They are SO time-consuming, and 2. They can be hard to shop for and keep track of!

Instead, I consider myself the queen (hence my name) of finding and creating high-protein, lower-calorie versions of some of my favorite foods! In fact, I originally earned my name, 'The Protein Snack Queen,' from my friends and clients for always having had a knack for discovering the latest and greatest high-protein snacks before they ever hit the mainstream. Over the last few years, I've compiled a growing list of these snacks, which you'll find at the very end of this cookbook!

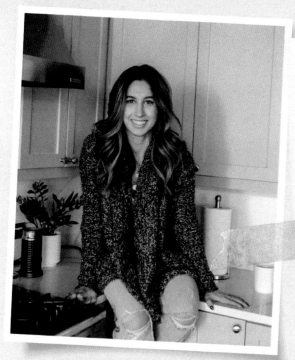

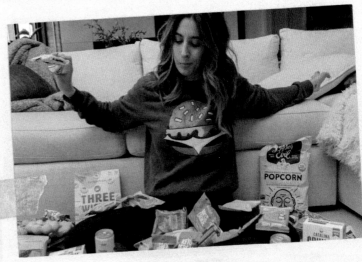

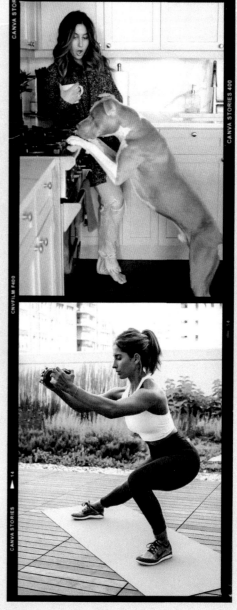

It was the compilation of that list that eventually led to the launch of 'The Protein Snack Queen' TikTok account!

Ultimately, my mission is to deliver authentic, approachable, and science-backed information to you at all times, empowering you with the knowledge to take control of your health & body! Eating healthily for sustainable fat loss doesn't have to be restrictive, boring, tasteless, time-consuming, or elaborate. My philosophy centers around finding the quickest, tastiest, and most protein-dense snacks and meals, without the extra, unnecessary calories.

This cookbook represents a new kind of guide – it's a shortcut for the busy, health-conscious individual who may not have the luxury of time to prepare a 40-ingredient recipe. Instead, it consists of meals assembled with healthy and delicious products, designed to cut your preparation time in half!

Creating this cookbook has been a true labor of love, and I hope the value you extract from it provides you with EMPOWERMENT, creativity, knowledge, and FUN! :)

Now that you're a part of the PSQ community, I'd love to hear about (and SEE!) your culinary creations! Feel free to get in touch or tag me on any of my social accounts!

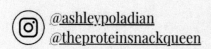
@ashleypoladian
@theproteinsnackqueen

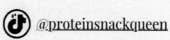
@proteinsnackqueen

But First, Some Context..

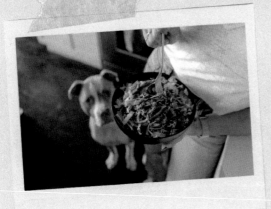 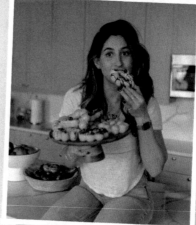

Knowledge is power, and I'd like to provide some helpful information to empower you with your food choices! Let's start by discussing macronutrients, also known as 'macros,' and explore why they are a frequent topic of conversation. Macronutrients are the primary nutrients that your body needs in relatively large quantities to function properly. They provide the energy (calories) for various body processes, support growth, and maintain bodily functions. There are three ESSENTIAL macronutrients:

Proteins
- Body Repair and Growth: Proteins are essential for building and repairing tissues, as they're made up of amino acids, the building blocks of the body.
- Types: There are essential amino acids (which we must obtain from our diet because the body cannot produce them) and non-essential amino acids (which the body can synthesize).
- Sources: Proteins can be found in meat, poultry, fish, dairy, legumes, nuts, and certain grains such as quinoa.
- Calories: Proteins provide about 4 calories per gram.
- Portion Size: A PALM generally determines your protein portion per meal. 1 palm equates to approximately 20-30g of protein.

Carbohydrates (Carbs)
- Source of Energy: Carbohydrates are the body's primary and preferred source of energy. Once consumed, they are broken down into glucose (sugar) and are either used immediately for energy or stored in the liver and muscles for later use.
- Types: Carbohydrates can be classified as simple (such as sugars found in fruits, milk, and candy) or complex (like those in whole grains, legumes, and starchy vegetables).
- Calories: Carbohydrates provide about 4 calories per gram.
- Portion Size: A FIST determines your vegetable portions, while a CUPPED HAND can generally determine your carb portion per meal. 1 cupped hand equates to approximately 20-30g of carbohydrates.

Fats (Lipids)
- nergy Storage: While carbs are the body's primary energy source, fats act as a secondary, more concentrated source of energy. They're essential for protecting organs, supporting cell growth, producing hormones, and absorbing certain vitamins.
- Types: There are several types of fats, including:
- Saturated Fats: Typically solid at room temperature, found in meats and dairy products.
- Unsaturated Fats: Usually liquid at room temperature, found in oils, nuts, and fish.
- Trans Fats: Often found in ultra-processed foods.
- Calories: Fats provide about 9 calories per gram, making them the most energy-dense macronutrient.
- Portion Size: A THUMB can generally determine your fat portion per meal. 1 thumb equates to approximately 7-12g of fat

So, Why Protein?

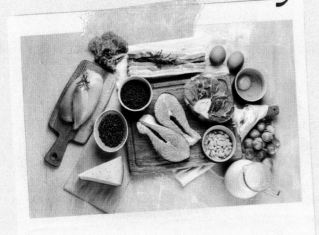 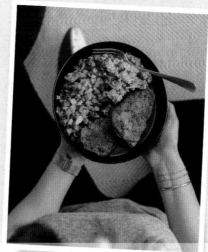

In addition to the primary macronutrients, the body also requires micronutrients, like vitamins and minerals, to operate. Micronutrients are used as co-factors in biological reactions and contain no energy or caloric value. However, they are important to consume for general health and well-being. You should never neglect including a variety of micronutrients in your food. The best way to be intentional about this is to always ensure you are consuming a colorful plate! Eating a variety of colors ensures you're consuming a diverse blend of micronutrients. This not only provides you with essential vitamins and minerals but also creates diversity in your gut. And yes, macronutrients have a whole host of micronutrients in them!

Now, why the heck am I obsessed with protein enough to call myself the Protein Snack Queen? Haha.

Iwork with busy people who care about losing body fat, building skeletal muscle, and living a strong and empowered life. For these reasons, protein is essential. For one, it's the most satiating macronutrient! For anyone trying to lose body fat, consuming a high-protein diet will keep you fuller for longer. You also burn more calories eating protein (it has a high thermic effect) than you do any other macronutrient because protein takes longer to digest.

Consuming a high-protein diet is essential for building lean tissue, a.k.a muscle! This is not only important for aesthetic reasons but imperative for overall well-being, especially as we age. As we grow older, our body's capacity to produce new proteins decreases. This necessitates a higher protein intake to maintain similar muscle protein synthesis. In fact, studies suggest you will need to enhance protein needs by 1% for each year over the age of 40. For example, a 50-year-old person might need to boost their protein consumption by 10% compared to the initial amount.

A high-protein diet also has a muscle-sparing effect! Not only is it beneficial to eat to stay full and burn more calories, but it's also key in reducing the loss of precious muscle when you're in a calorie deficit. A calorie deficit occurs when you consume fewer calories than your body uses for energy, ultimately leading to fat loss. Studies using higher protein diets have been shown to produce more fat loss and spare more lean muscle mass compared to calorie-equated diets lower in protein.

The development and preservation of lean tissue is one of the most important health hacks of our time. Aside from the pancreas and liver, muscles are the most important organ to regulate glucose---and glucose regulation is IMPERATIVE for controlling disease risk. Build muscle with protein because the more muscle you have, the better you can store glucose with less insulin.

The current Recommended Daily Allowance (RDA) for protein consumption is 0.8g of protein per kg of body weight. However, according to more recent literature and several experts in the field, minimum protein requirements fall within the 0.8-1.2g per lb of lean body mass range. For someone engaging in strength training who wants to OPTIMIZE muscle development, the target could be anywhere between 1.6-2.2g/kg of lean body mass (LBM). Protein intake upwards of 3g per kg of body weight has been tested without adverse effects in healthy individuals. To simplify this, I usually aim for 1g of protein per lb of body weight, adjusting more or less depending on the individual and their experience with eating a higher-protein diet. If you're new to a high-protein regimen, consider starting on the lower end and gradually building up as you develop a routine for consuming more protein.

Along with TOTAL protein intake, protein source and quality also matter. There are many different types of protein, with animal-based protein being one of the most optimal sources we as humans can absorb and process, especially for muscle development. Research has indicated that plant proteins are generally less optimal than animal proteins for muscular development. This is a VERY NUANCED topic, however, and there are no absolutes.

Protein in whole plant sources like beans and legumes is typically not as high in quality due to the lack of bioavailability (50%-70% because it's bound up in fibrous plant material), making it harder to digest and absorb. Plant sources of protein are also found to be lower in branched-chain amino acids, essential amino acids, and the amino acid leucine, which positively affects muscle protein synthesis and muscle mass.

The caveat, however, is that it is still VERY possible to build muscle on a plant-based diet, especially if you are utilizing plant protein isolate powders. Someone following a plant-based diet will need to consume MORE plant proteins in volume, and often MORE CALORIES, to absorb the same amount of protein and amino acids found in animal varieties. Since plant protein sources also contain carbohydrates, those on a plant-based diet usually consume more carbohydrates as a result. Animal proteins, on the other hand, typically have very little carbohydrate content.

Ultimately, intent matters -- if your intent is to build the most muscle possible, or preserve the most muscle possible during a calorie deficit, then favoring animal protein may be a better option. If your intent is to eat enough protein to be healthy, and possibly build some muscle, you are perfectly fine eating plant-based proteins.

The variations of proteins listed on the next page are outlined by how much protein per gram the respective food contains. As you move down the list, you'll find that foods go from "all protein" to "mostly protein, some fat" to "protein and fat." This is relevant because the top half of the list gives you more protein per calorie than the bottom half. If your goal is weight loss, consider including proteins from the top of the list MORE often than those from the bottom. Again, fats are great & incredibly important, but relying on fatty proteins every day isn't the most efficient approach to a calorie deficit. You may even consider sourcing your fats from other flavorful options, such as avocado or nuts.

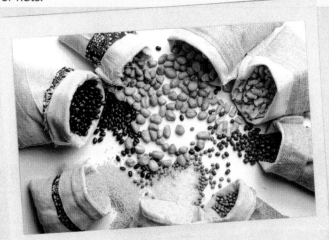
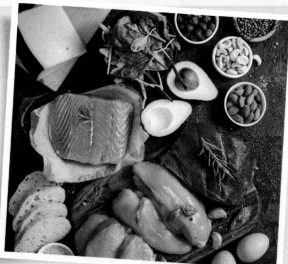

Protein-Rich Foods

In order of caloric density, starting with the least calories _PER 100 G_ to most, roughly:

Egg Whites - 52 cal / 11g protein

Fat Free Yogurt - 60 cal/ 8g protein

Cod - 82 cal/ 18g protein

Crab - 90 cal / 19g protein

Shrimp - 99 cal / 24g protein

1 Scoop of Whey Protein (30 g) - 121 cal / 30g protein

Duck Breast (no skin) - 123 cal / 24g protein

Tilapia - 129 cal/ 26g protein

Seitan - 130 cal/ 25g protein

Tofu - 145 cal / 15g protein

Yellowtail Sashimi - 146 cal / 26g protein

Fat-Free Cheese - 148 calories / 23g protein

99% Lean Ground Chicken - 160 cal / 26g protein

99% Lean Ground Turkey - 160 cal/26g protein

Chicken Breast (no skin) - 165 cal / 26 g protein

Turkey Breast (no skin) - 165 cal /26g protein

Chicken/Turkey/Duck - Dark Meat: 180 cal/23g protein

Duck Breast (with skin) - 202 cal/ 24g protein

Eye of Round Roast Steak - 145 calories /5g protein

Sirloin Tip - 150 calories / 27g protein

Top Round - 180 calories / 28g protein

Bottom Round Roast - 160 cal / 23g protein

Top SIrloin Steak - 200 cal/ 20g protein

96% lean ground Beef - 140 cal/ 24g protein

Whole Eggs -150 cal / 12g protein

Salmon- 146-200 cal/ 21g protein

Sardines - 208 cal/ 24g protein

Bacon - 540 cal/ 37g protein'

Lentils - Protein & Carbohydtrates- 25-30g in 1 cup

Beans - Protein & Carbohydtrates - 15-20g in 1 cup

Nutritional Yeast - 8g protein in 2 T

Hemp Seeds- protein & fat - 11g protein per 30g

Chia Seeds - Protein &Fat- 5g protein per 30g

Quinoa - protein & carbohydtrates - 8g protein per 1 cup

Peas- protein & carbohydtrates - 4g protein per 1.2/ cup

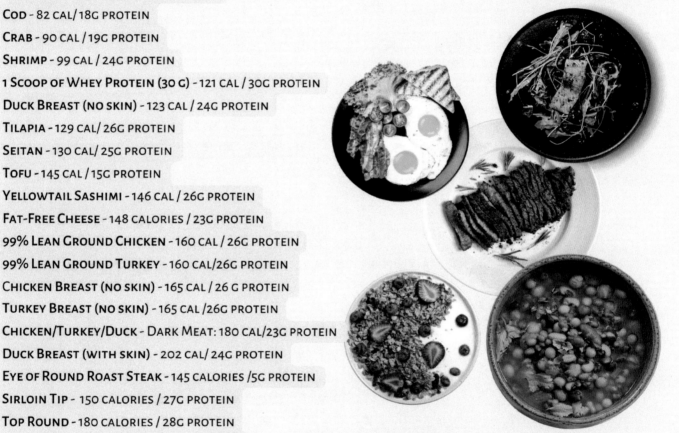

Nutritional Priorities for Fat Loss

1. Calorie (Energy) Balance and Adherence.

Energy balance is simply a matter of calories in versus calories out. You cannot lose body fat without being in a negative energy balance, also known as a calorie deficit. THIS IS RULE NUMBER ONE! Consuming fewer calories than you are expending is theoretically simple but can be complex in practice. Many online calculators can provide a ballpark range of calories, but the best method is to track your normal daily intake for 1-2 weeks, assess your weight changes, and adjust your calories accordingly. If you're serious about this process, hiring a coach can guide you more effectively and ensure adherence to a plan. Without adherence, there is no plan.

2. Protein & Fiber Intake.

We've already covered why protein is crucial for fat loss & satiety. Fiber, too, has a thermogenic effect similar to protein while improving satiety. Since fiber adds "bulk," it is filling and aids digestion. It's a misconception that fiber is calorie-free, so please, let's stop subtracting fiber from carbs to count only net carbs :)

3. Self Monitoring.

You measure what you manage and don't manage what you don't measure. Evidence strongly supports that active monitoring correlates with successful, sustained weight loss. Studies show that individuals weighing themselves daily or tracking food intake tend to maintain weight more effectively. This continuous feedback loop fosters a disciplined and responsive approach to weight management.

4. Carbs and Fats.

Both carbohydrates and fats are essential to the fat-loss process. Carbohydrates, our primary energy source, are vital for fueling our daily activities, especially during fat loss. Insufficient energy can hinder workouts and fat loss. Fats are necessary for nutrient absorption and hormone regulation, both crucial for fat loss and muscle building.

4. Protein Distribution.

Consuming enough protein throughout the day is essential, but distributing your intake evenly can optimize fat loss and muscle development. Since the body can't store surplus protein, maintaining amino acids in the blood becomes vital during a calorie deficit. Proper distribution ensures that enough amino acids are always available for muscle building. Assuming you're eating about 4 meals a day, aim for 25g-45g of protein per meal.

Behavioral Priorities for Fat Loss

Stress Management.
SStress represents a shift in our physiological condition, a reaction to what our bodies perceive as a threatening situation. Governed by the autonomic nervous system—which is continually active—our body is constantly striving to strike a balance between states of calm and stress. This intricate system is responsible for managing our physiological responses, ensuring an equilibrium between relaxation and alertness.Understanding and managing stress in the context of your physical well-being is an essential aspect of health. It directly affects not only mental clarity but also various bodily functions, which can subsequently impact your goals for losing body fat or building muscle

Quality Sleep.
Sleep stands as one of the most vital and often overlooked tools in our arsenal for assisting with fat loss. Most individuals either a) don't get sufficient sleep, or b) experience poor sleep quality. The significance of sleep extends far beyond mere recovery; it's also essential for maintaining adherence to our health routines. Inadequate sleep leads to changes in our hunger hormones, specifically causing a decrease in the feeling of fullness and satisfaction, making us more prone to overeating. This physiological reaction, coupled with elevated hunger levels due to poor sleep, forms a particularly detrimental scenario when it comes to adhering to our health and wellness goals.

Resistance/Strength Training.
Strength training is quite simply the fountain of youth! Some key benefits of strength training include improvements in cognitive and mental health, increased bone density, the development of lean muscle, increased strength (which is especially important as we age), and enhanced energy, confidence, and self-empowerment. For fat loss, however, strength training is the mechanism through which we build quality tissue like muscle because protein cannot build muscle without resistance training. In addition, as stated before, strength work will not only help you increase your energy expenditure but also help you preserve lean muscle when you're losing body fat. This preservation of lean muscle contributes to the "toned" look that many people desire.

Movement.
I'I'm grouping movement separately from strength training on purpose to encompass all the movement that happens outside of the gym. This includes NEAT, also known as Non-Exercise Activity Thermogenesis, and walking. NEAT represents all the unintentional movements you make. When you're simply standing, numerous muscles across your body are engaged to maintain your posture, even though you might not be consciously controlling them. NEAT contributes to approximately 25% of the overall energy expenditure for the average person. However, it's worth noting that this percentage can vary significantly among individuals. Walking can arguably be grouped separately from NEAT since it is usually done intentionally. Regardless, it is important to keep yourself moving throughout the day. I always like to tell clients that exercising is only 1 hour out of 24, so you shouldn't rely on it solely for weight loss. Instead, if you move for several hours throughout the day, you increase your energy expenditure significantly, ultimately encouraging a higher probability of fat loss

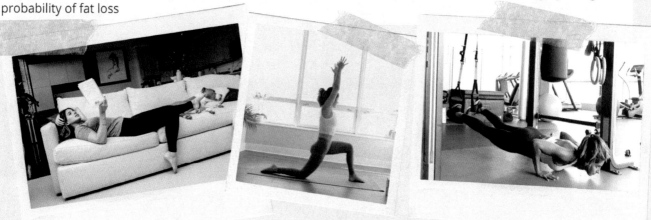

But Before Any of That....

The single most important thing you can do to lose body fat, build muscle, or achieve ANY goal, really, is...

DESIGN A NEW IDENTITY & EMBODY THAT IDENTITY. (Thanks, James Clear!)

We live our lives through a series of personal habits. Our habits are developed by our actions, which are developed by our feelings, which are in turn developed by our thoughts and beliefs. Put simply, your current behaviors are a reflection of your current self-concept, or the type of person you think you are. How you perceive who you are, what you're capable of, and what you deserve has a direct correlation with the choices you make in your life. Achieving any goal, then, is highly dependent on how you embody the qualities of the person who WOULD achieve that goal.

If being STRONG is your goal, identify characteristics in the strong people in your life. Choose some of the most admirable and begin to embody them. If being confident is a goal, identify characteristics of some of the most confident people in your life, and embody the ones that speak to you. If fat loss is your goal, identify some of the healthiest people in your life and choose to embody some of their most admirable characteristics related to being healthy and fit.

Objectively speaking, losing body fat is actually a relatively straightforward endeavor, but it never feels straightforward because we're human, nuanced, and emotional. If you can hack your self-identity by erasing the self-sabotaging limiting beliefs and creating new, affirming, and productive ones, you will be primed to not only achieve your goals but thrive and sustain them.

Let's get to work! 💪

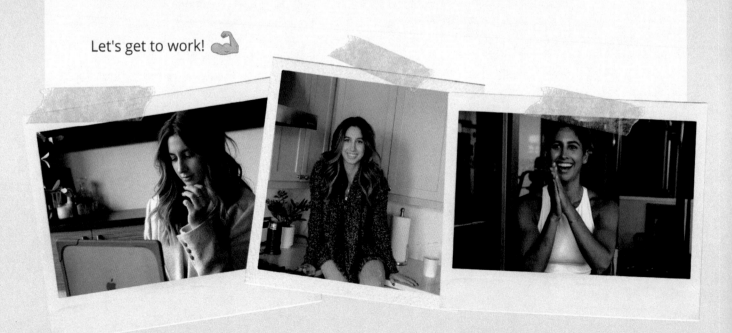

Tips for Staying Consistent

- **The less variety you have in your meals** from day to day, the easier it will be to stick to your diet goals. Variety often leads to a higher likelihood of error.
- If fat loss is your goal, **eat on small plates** to make your meals look larger.
- **Plan (and prep for bonus points) your meals ahead of time,** so you're prepared and have visibility into your options. It's like budgeting!
- **Practice portion control!** Don't eat snacks directly from the container or bag. Scoop out a predetermined amount and place it into a bowl or onto a plate. If you eat straight from the package, you're more likely to overeat! I've listed helpful portion guides on a previous page.
- Time your meals and snacks strategically. If you enjoy snacking in the evenings, save your carbs for then. Consuming higher protein foods earlier helps save calories for later.
- **Shop with the PROTEIN to CALORIE RATIO in mind!** Take a glance at a product's calories, drop the last number, and aim for the protein content to be as close to that number as possible. Being within 20% is a good rule of thumb. If the protein content exceeds the edited calorie number, you've found a WINNER! This equates to having 10% of calories come from protein. (Example: 250 calories becomes 25. Aim for 25 grams of protein.
- **Make tempting food harder to acquire.** Keep tempting foods away and delete food delivery apps if you're prone to impulse ordering.
- **Watch your portions.** If you crave a cookie, buy ONE, not a box.
- **Be mindful of serving sizes and portions!** Food labels can deceive, so it's crucial to measure food accurately.
- If you eat something that doesn't fit your macros, IT'S OKAY. **CONSISTENCY matters most.** Focus on your overall pattern rather than occasional slip-ups.
- Remember, **our biology drives us to seek food** – an evolutionary trait that doesn't always align with modern lifestyles. Cutting back on food may increase hunger hormones, leading you to think about food more often. Instead of resisting this natural urge, align your environment with your goals by implementing the strategies listed above. :)"

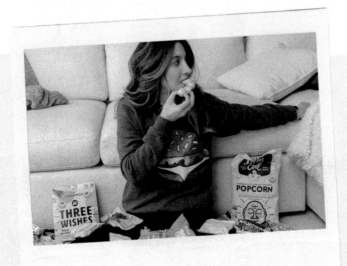

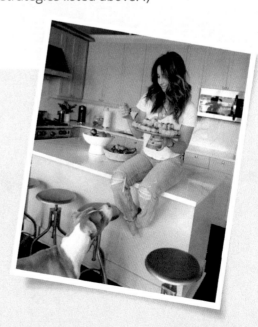

Tips for Staying Consistent

If you're dining out.....

- **Plan Ahead.** The more prepared you are, the better your chances of success. Determine where you're going and look at the menu ahead of time to choose some menu options that you believe may fit within your goals. This almost always looks like a protein-centered dish where the protein is the star--- not pasta or pizza with protein in it. Think about a chicken dish, a lean steak dish, a white fish dish, scallops, mussels..etc.

- **Choose something other than fried food.** Fried food is just not good for you, and it certainly isn't great if you're trying to watch your caloric intake. It's impossible to know how much fat is in a deep-fried dish, and it's usually much more than we think. We know fat is double the calories per gram than carbohydrates or protein, so having a lot of it will increase your calorie intake FAST.

- **Ask for steamed vegetables instead of sauteed.** Sauteed vegetables as a side may seem healthy but restaurants usually don't hold back on butter and oil to flavor a vegetable dish. Ask for steamed vegetables to avoid the added calories from the extra oil.

- **Skip the bread or any heavy apps prior to the entree.** You don't need to be consuming anything more than your meal unless you REALLY want to.

- **Share plates whenever possible.** This is a psychology play. If you're sharing your food, you not only don't eat all of it, you're less inclined to eat a lot because you're typically trying to be polite.

- **Have a dessert strategy.** Determine if the dessert on the menu is desirable enough, or if the company you're with even wants dessert. If yes to both, then draw boundaries around how much dessert you'll have. 1-2 bites is what I suggest.

- **Never say you CAN'T have anything.** Always remember that you are in control. It is never about restriction, just preference and moderation. You are choosing the healthier choices in every moment-- that is true power.

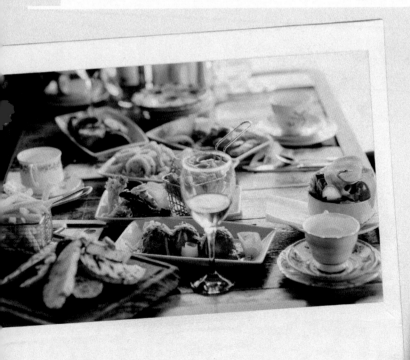

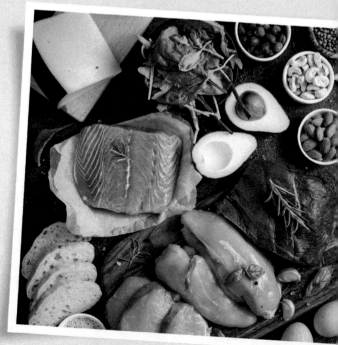

Kitchen Tools You'll Want

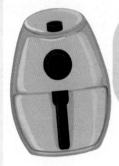

An Air Fryer! I use an air fryer a lot in my recipes, and I truly believe they are one of the best purchases you can make for your kitchen! I use a Dreo & love how portable it is--- I just tuck it into a kitchen cabinet when I'm done! I'll offer baking alternatives to air fryer recipes, but do yourself a favor and get an air fryer if you don't have one!

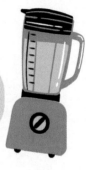

A blender! I use a small one (the Beast) because I hate bringing out the big toys. It comes in handy when I need to blend something small...plus, it's easy to clean and store!

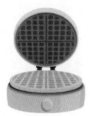

TThere are two recipes in this cookbook that call for the use of a waffle maker. I jumped on the waffle maker train to make protein pancakes easier and more approachable. If you're a protein pancake enthusiast but hate the process, mess, and cleanup,consider getting a waffle maker!

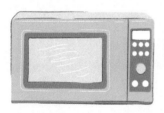

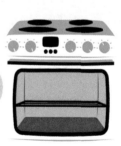

A microwave and an oven! This is self-explanatory and I'm almost certain you have these! :)

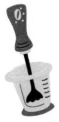

If you know me, you know I love a good immersion blend! This tool is such a hack and so much easier to manage than a blender. Still, a blender has its place-- but an immersion blender is a GREAT kitchen tool. You'll want it to whip up some cottage cheese! ;)

Common Ingredients to Have on Hand...

- Lean Meat like Chicken, Turkey, and Rotisserie Chicken, 96% lean beef
- Reduced Fat Shredded Cheese
- Low Fat/Fat-Free Cottage Cheese
- Low Fat/Fat-Free Greek Yogurt
- Protein Powder of choice, usually Vanilla or Chocolate
- No sugar added Milk - Plant or regular
- All-purpose flour
- High Protein Wraps of choice
- Lite Mayo
- Ketchup
- Sriracha
- Zero Calorie Sweetener of choice
- Monk Fruit sweetener
- Monk Fruit Syrup
- Egg whites
- Eggs
- Turkey Bacon
- Avocado oil
- Coconut Aminos or Soy Sauce
- Pastas & Rice - Protein Pasta & Hearts of Palm
- Vegetables like cucumbers, peppers, tomatos

My snack and product catalog is at the end of this cookbook!

Table Of Contents

BREAKFAST

Nutrient Dense Shake..1
Greek Yogurt Cereal Bowl.......................................2
Extra High-Protein Scrambled Eggs.................3
Hearty Sausage & Eggs Scramble.....................4
Super Savory Omelette...5
Eggwhite Sausage & Cheese Sandwich................6
Fajita Egg Muffin Cups...7
Scallion Pancake Breakfast Pizza.....................8
High-Protein French Toast Bites........................9
Breakfast French Toast Roll-Ups...................10
High Protein Breakfast Sandwich....................11
Bagel & Lox 12
Cheesy Egg Bagel..13
Chocolate Banana Chia Pudding......................14
Strawberry Chia Pudding...................................15
Strawberry Vanilla Yogurt Toast....................16
High Protein Carrot Cake Overnight Oats...........17

LUNCH & DINNER

High-Protein Chicken Salad/Wrap.....................18
Easy Turkey BLT Wrap..19
Cheesy Chicken Taquito...20
Lazy Chicken Caesar Wrap...................................21
Lazy Buffalo Chicken Wrap.................................22
7-Min Spinach Dip Chickenburger Sandwich..23
Southwest Style Chicken Wrap........................24
Turkey Pinwheels...25
Taco Pinwheels..26
Cheeseburger Eggrolls..27
Pizza Roll Ups...28
5-minute Quesadillas...29
BBQ Chicken Jicama Tacos..................................30
Ashley's Favorite Salmon Wrap........................31
Cottage Cheese Bruschetta Toast....................32
Greek-inspired Chicken Hummus Wrap 33
Cheeseburger Quesadillas...................................34

Table Of Contents

LUNCH & DINNER (cont.)

Trader Joe's Gyro Sandwich.....................................35
Greek Cottage Cheese Bowl....................................36
Spring Roll in a Bowl...37
Ashley's Egg Salad..38
Cheeseburger Bowl...39
Cucumber Chili Crunch Salad..................................40
Feta and Cheddar Stuffed Mini Peppers...............41
Hamburger Meatloaf Bites.....................................42
Korean-Style Vegetable Pancakes.........................43
Greek-Inspired Chicken Patties 44
Cobb Salad..45
Beet & Feta Salad...46
Asian-Inspired Kelp Noodle Salad.........................47
Edamame Honey Sesame Chicken Salad...............48
Elote Salad..49
Cucumber Ginger Sashimi Salad............................50
High-Protein Low-Carb Pasta Salad......................51
Middle Eastern Beef & Yogurt Pasta.....................52
Beef-less Stuffed Peppers......................................53
Spinach & Ricotta Stuffed Chicken........................54
Single Serving Low Carb Lasagna..........................55
High-Protein Mac and Cheese................................56
Low-Carb Cauliflower "Mac & Cheese"..................57
Low Carb High-Protein Alfredo Pasta....................58
My Favorite Healthy Meatloaf................................59
My Favorite Low-Carb Bean-less Chili...................60
Low-Calorie Spring Rolls & Peanut Sauce.............61
Sushi Cups...62
Easy Sushi Wrap...63
Waffle Crispy Rice...64
Lavash Bread Pizza...65
White Sauce Lavash Pizza......................................66
Crispy Salmon & Cheese Taco................................67
Trader Joe's Mediterranean Bowl..........................68
Taco Casserole..69
Sweet Pepper Nachos...70
Cilantro Lime Shrimp Tacos...................................71
Beef Tostada...72
Taco Bowl..73

Table Of Contents

SMALL DISHES, SIDES & DIPS

Mediterranean Side Salad...74
High-Protein Hashbrown Fritters......................75
Protein Naan Bread...76
Protein Garlic Cheesy Bread............................77
High-Protein Low-Carb Jicama Fries....................78
Crispy Carrots..79
Buffalo Chicken Dip..80
Spinach Artichoke & Chicken Dip......................81
Elote Dip..82
Red Pepper Cottage CHeese Dip........................83
Turkey Bacon Wrapped Stuffed Dates..................84
Peach & "Burrata" Toast.....................................85
Everything But the Bagel Lox Roll.........................86

SWEET TREATS

High-Protein Tiramisu...87
High-Protein Chocolate Strawberry Crepe...........88
High Protein PB&J Tortilla....................................89
Birthday Cake Protein Waffles............................90
Protein Strawberry Cheesecake............................91
Apple Pie Mug Cake...92
High-Protein Edible Cookie Dough....................93
Protein Fruit Bake Crumble..............................94
Elvis Dumplings...95
Protein Chocolate Peanut Butter Balls...................96
Protein S'mores Bowl..97
Vanilla Ricotta Blintz...98
Banana Cream Pie Bowl......................................99
High-Protein Monkey Bread.................................100

SNACKS & PRODUCTS CATALOG

Breakfast Products 101,102
Lunch & Dinner Products (Pasta)...........................103
Lunch & Dinner Products (Rice/Frozen)...............104
Lunch & Dinner Products (Breads/Tortillas).........105
Lunch & Dinner Products (Pizzas/Dressings).........106
Snack Products..107
Desserts & Candy 108
Icecream...109
Drinks & Protein Powders................................110

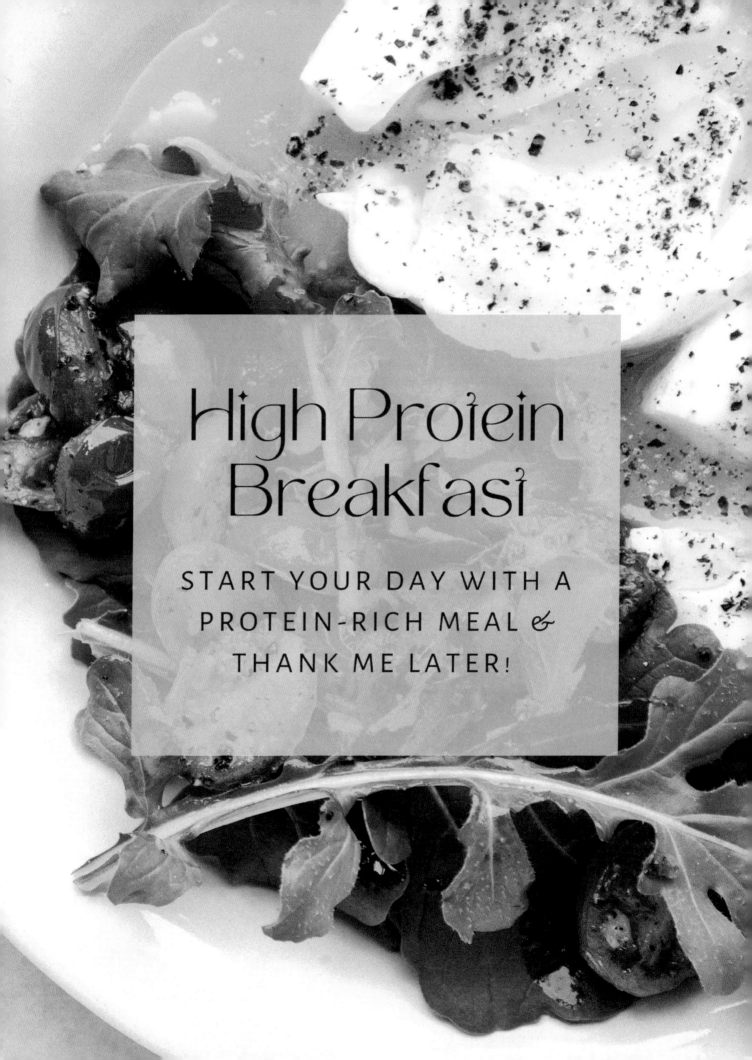

High Protein Breakfast

START YOUR DAY WITH A
PROTEIN-RICH MEAL &
THANK ME LATER!

Nutrient-Dense Protein Shake ✓

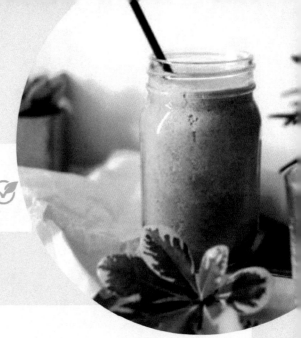

SERVINGS: 1 PREPPING TIME: 2 MIN COOKING TIME: 0 MIN

INGREDIENTS

- 1/2 cup blueberries
- 1 scoop (20g of protein) vanilla protein powder
- 1/2 cup (120g) unsweetened almond milk
- 1/4 banana
- 1 T PB2 Peanut Butter Powder
- 1 Scoop of Clean Simple Eats Super Greens (or any other green powder).
- 1 cup frozen broccoli
- 1 cup frozen spinach

PROTEINSNACKQUEEN gets you 10% off!

DIRECTIONS

1. Blend all together and enjoy!

Calories: 270 | Carbohydrate: 22g | Protein: 33g | Fat: 5 grams

Greek Yogurt Cereal Bowl ✅

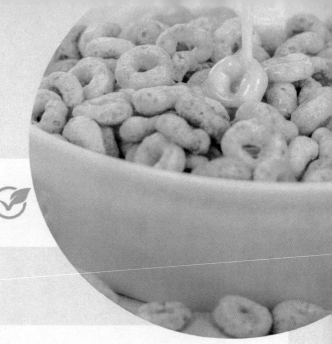

SERVINGS: 1   PREPPING TIME: 2 MIN   COOKING TIME: 0 MIN

INGREDIENTS

- 1 & 1/2 cup 0% Greek Yogurt (200g)
- 1T Reduced Sugar Raspberry Preserves
- 15g (or 1/2 oz) <u>Three Wishes Cinnamon Protein Cereal</u> (or any other cinnamon protein cereal!)

DIRECTIONS

1. Mix greek yogurt with Raspberry Preserves
2. Add Cereal. Mix and enjoy!

Calories: 200 | Carbohydrate: 24 g | Protein: 24g | Fat: 1g

Extra High-Protein Scrambled Eggs

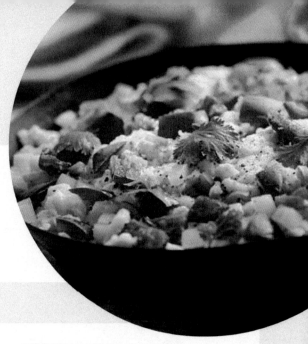

SERVINGS: 1   PREPPING TIME: 5 MIN   COOKING TIME: 5-10 MIN

INGREDIENTS

- Oil Spray
- 2 whole eggs
- 1/4 cup liquid egg whites
- 1/2 cup fat free or low fat cottage cheese
- 1/4 cup oil-free Pico De Gallo
- Salt, pepper, onion and garlic powder to taste

If you don't like cottage cheese in eggs, use an additional 1/4 cup of egg whites and 1 oz of lite cheese instead. This substitution will result in a nutritional content of 280 calories, 34g of protein, 6g of carbs, and 14g of fat.

DIRECTIONS

1. Spray your pan with 1 spray of oil
2. Crack two eggs into the pan and scramble, keeping heat to medium-low
3. Add 1/4 cup liquid egg whites and stir
4. Add 1/2 cup blended fat free or low fat cottage cheese
5. Cover pan and let eggs cook until white, stir occasionally until desired consistency is achieved!
6. Add 1/2 cup fresh salsa + salt and pepper & cover for 1-2 more minutes.

Calories: 255 | Carbohydrate: 9g | Protein: 32 g | Fat: 10g

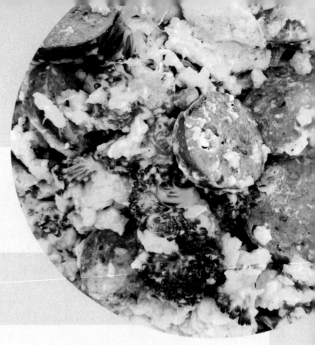

Hearty Sausage and Eggs Scramble

SERVINGS: 1   PREPPING TIME: 5 MIN   COOKING TIME: 8 MIN

INGREDIENTS

- 1 organic <u>chicken sausage</u> link, sliced 1/4 inch thick
- 2 eggs
- 1-2 sprays of Avocado Oil
- 1 cup chopped broccoli florets
- 1/4 small onion, chopped small
- 1 clove garlic, minced
- Sea salt and black pepper to taste

DIRECTIONS

1. Warm oil in a skillet over medium heat.
2. Add the sliced sausage, broccoli, onion, and garlic to the skillet, and cook for 5 minutes, stirring occasionally.
3. In a separate bowl, whisk the eggs, then add them to the skillet along with salt and pepper.
4. Stir the mixture until the eggs are cooked through.
5. Remove from heat and serve warm.

Calories: 280 | Carbohydrate: 11g | Protein: 30g | Fat: 13g

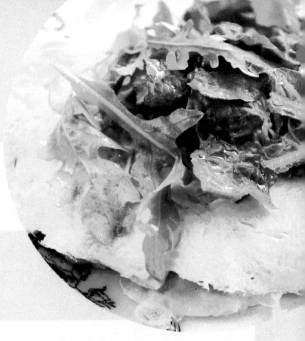

Super Savory Omelette

SERVINGS: 1   PREP TIME: 5 MINUTES   COOKING TIME: 5 MINUTES

INGREDIENTS

- 2 large eggs
- Salt and pepper to taste
- 1 spray avocado oil
- 2 tbsp (8 g) red onions, chopped
- Handful of spinach or arugula
- 2 tbsp (28 g/ 1 oz) goat cheese
- 2 slices of organic turkey bacon, sliced

DIRECTIONS

1. In a bowl, whisk eggs with goat cheese until fluffy.
2. In a small skillet, heat olive oil.
3. Add red onions and turkey to the skillet. Cook for 2-3 minutes, then remove from heat.
4. Add eggs to the skillet and cook for 1-2 minutes, or until the sides begin to lift from the bottom. Flip the eggs.
5. Top with the cooked onions and turkey mixture. Cook for an additional 30 seconds - 1 minute, or until the eggs are cooked through.
6. Fold the eggs in half, remove from heat, and enjoy!

Calories: 310 | Carbohydrate: 4g | Protein: 31 | Fat: 19g

Eggwhite, Sausage & Cheese Sandwich

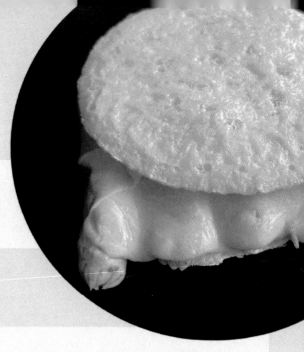

SERVINGS: 1   PREPPING TIME: 5-7 MIN   COOKING TIME: 1 MIN

INGREDIENTS

- 2 Good Food Made Simple Egg White Patties OR Cooked Egg Whites made into discs before hand (think like pancakes)
- Lite/Reduced Fat Cheese Slices (Tis,Kraft, Sargento)
- 1 Sliced Chicken Sausage (Tjs, Bilinski's -- under 130 calories)
- Everything But the Bagel Seasoning

DIRECTIONS

1. If you're making your egg white patties from scratch, pour egg whites into a muffin tin or a small pan. Bake at 350°F for 15 minutes beforehand.
2. Using 2 patties, slice chicken sausage into thin slivers and lay on top of the egg white patty.
3. Place a slice of low-fat cheese on the sausages resting on the egg white patty.
4. Toss into a microwave for 45 seconds to melt the cheese. Sprinkle with Everything But The Bagel Seasoning.
5. Place the second egg white patty on top.

Calories: 240 | Carbohydrate: 7g | Protein: 31g | Fat: 10g

Fajita Egg Muffin Cups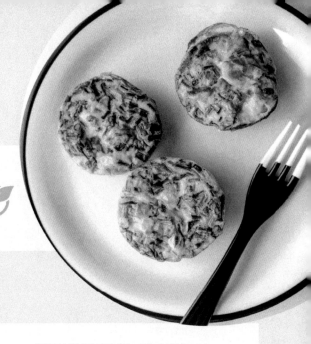

SERVINGS: 1   PREPPING TIME: 5 MIN   COOKING TIME: 25 MIN

INGREDIENTS

- 3 large whole eggs
- 1 cup egg whites (or 7 large egg white)
- 1/2 cup reduced shredded cheddar cheese. Fat free reduces calories more!
- 1 cup frozen spinach
- 1 cup chopped bell peppers (can use frozen pre-chopped)
- 6 T fresh pico de gallo salsa (I love Trader Joe's!)
- Salt & Pepper

DIRECTIONS

1. Preheat oven to 375 degrees F.
2. Spray the muffin pan with a slight spray of oil or butter.
3. Plop chopped bell peppers, spinach, pico de gallo, & cheese in each muffin cup.
4. Combine eggs and egg whites & beat together.
5. Pour mixture evenly across all muffin cup slots.
6. Bake for about 25-30 minutes
7. Let cool, refrigerate/ freeze, or enjoy right away!

Makes 9 muffins: Calories per muffin:
Calories: 60, Carbohydrate: 1g, Protein: 7g | Fat: 3 grams

Scallion Pancake Breakfast Pizza 🌱

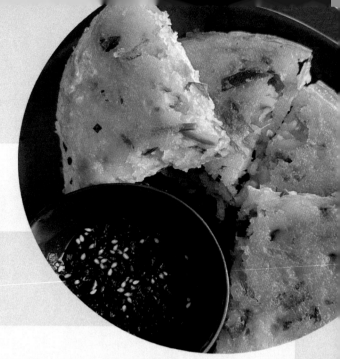

SERVINGS: 1	PREPPING TIME: 5 MIN	COOKING TIME: 10 MIN

INGREDIENTS

- 1 Scallion Pancake from Trader Joe's (Pa Jeon)
- 9 T liquid eggwhites
- 1 whole egg
- 2 T coconut aminos

Dipping Sauce:

1/4 cup Coconut Aminos

Furikake Seasoning

DIRECTIONS

1. Heat your scallion pancake in the microwave for 1-2 minutes to defrost.
2. In a small bowl, whisk together egg whites, an egg, and 2 T coconut aminos.
3. Grease a small pan over medium heat and pour the egg mixture over. Cover with a lid to let the eggs partially cook.
4. Once mostly cooked, place the scallion pancake on top of the eggs and let cook, covered, for another couple of minutes.
5. Once the eggs are hard, flip the pancake with the eggs so the pancake side is facing down on the pan. Let the pancake cook through & get crispy.
6. Once cooked, set on a plate and slice like a pizza. Use sauce for dipping!

Calories: 344 | Carbohydrate: 28g | Protein: 26g | Fat: 14g

High-Protein French Toast Bites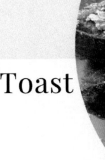

SERVINGS: ABOUT 12 BITES   PREPPING TIME: 10-15 MIN   COOKING TIME: 10 MIN

INGREDIENTS

- 1 <u>ROYO BREAD</u> Burger Bun (or any other burger bun)
- 1 scoop of cinnamon protein powder (I used GAINFUL, but you can use your favorite. You can also use Vanilla and add cinnamon!)
- 1/4 cup milk
- 1 egg
- Cinnamon powder to taste

Cinnamon Brown Sugar:

- 3 T Lakanto Golden
- Cinnamon powder

DIRECTIONS

1. Start by cutting the bun into small pieces face down
2. Create a batter with 1 egg, 1 scoop protein powder, milk, and cinnamon.
3. Warm a pan with oil.
4. Dunk each piece of bread in batter, then cook on pan til golden colored
5. Remove from eat and dunk each in cinnamon sugar!
6. Follow with some Lakanto Maple Syrup as desired!

Calories: 400 | Carbohydrate: 44g | Protein: 36g | Fat: 9g

Breakfast French Toast Roll-Up

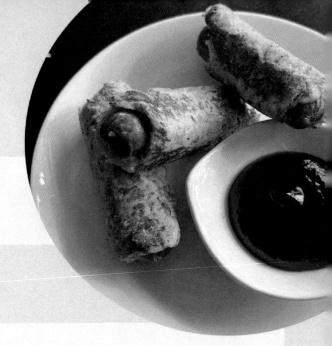

SERVINGS: 3 ROLLS   PREPPING TIME: 5-7 MIN   COOKING TIME: 5 MIN

INGREDIENTS

- 3 slices of bread, crust removed
- 1 Slice of low fat cheddar cheese
- 3 Mini breakfast sausages (used the Maple Chicken from Trader Joe's)
- 1 egg, beaten
- Avocado oil spray
- Optional dipping: ketchup, maple syrup

DIRECTIONS

1. Remove the crusts from the bread and flatten the bread gently.
2. Whisk one egg in a bowl.
3. Dip one side of bread into the bowl with the egg mixture.
4. Placing the wet side down, place a sausage and 1/3 slice of cheese on one end of the bread.
5. Roll tightly & repeat 2 more times.
6. Spray some avocado oil in a skillet and heat with medium heat.
7. Place rolls seam-side down on the skillet to cook edges together.
8. Once golden brown, remove from heat and enjoy with some ketchup!

Calories for one roll: 150 | Carbohydrate: 15g | Protein: 12g | Fat: 5g

High-Protein Breakfast Sandwich

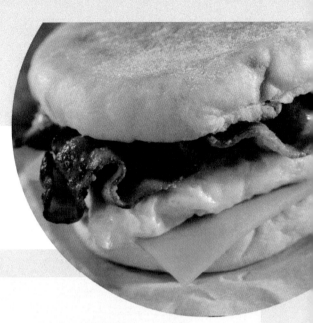

SERVINGS: 1	PREPPING TIME: 0 MIN	COOKING TIME: 10 MIN

INGREDIENTS

- 1/2 tsp butter or cooking spray
- 1 Good Food Made SImple Eggwhite Patty or 1/2 c egg whites
- 1 English Muffin or 2 slices of low calorie bread (I love Royo)
- Low fat cheese of choice
- 2 slices of turkey bacon

Excellent Alternative:

Red's Eggwich from Costco (video)

DIRECTIONS

1. Warm butter or oil in a skillet over medium heat.
2. Place bread or English muffin face down to cook.
3. Place egg white patty on pan or in a separate small pan; cook egg whites.
4. Place a slice of cheese over egg whites and cover pan so cheese melts.
5. Once cooked, add patty melt onto one piece of bread.
6. Add 1-2 pieces of cooked turkey bacon.
7. Cover with the second piece of bread.

Calories: 292 | Carbohydrate: 26g | Protein: 29g | Fat: 8g

Bagel & Lox

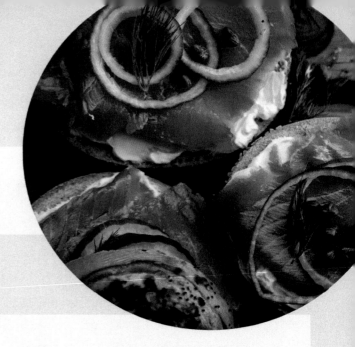

SERVINGS:1   PREPPING TIME: 5 MIN   COOKING TIME: 1 MIN

INGREDIENTS

- 1 Bagel of Choice (see list of my favorites below)
- 2 slices of Everything but the Bagel Smoked Salmon from Trader Joe's or any Smoked Salmon of choice
- Everything but the Bagel Greek Style Yogurt dip (sub with whipped cottage cheese or Greek yogurt seasoned with Everything seasoning!)
- Optional: Sliced cucumbers, sliced onions, capers, dill

DIRECTIONS

1. Warm your bagel.
2. Add 1 serving of Everything but the Bagel dip (or greek yogurt, cream cheese)
3. Slice smoked salmon slices in half and place on the bagel
4. Season with more Everything Seasoning
5. Optional to add sliced cucumber and red onion!

- ROYO Low Carb, HIGH FIBER Bread - [1 slice - 30 cal,, 11g Fiber] CODE: PROTEINSNACKQUEEN
- ROYO Low Carb Everything Bagel - [1 bagel- 80 cal] CODE: PROTEINSNACKQUEEN
- Gluten Free PAGEL 250 calories - 4g protein, 43g carbs, 8g fat
- The Better Bagel - 160 calories, 26g protein, 40g carbs, 2g fat
- Zero Carb Bagel - 90 calories, 14g protein, 14g carbs, 4 g fat

Calories for 1 whole bagel: 330 | Carbohydrate: 41g | **Protein: 23g** | Fat: 13g

Cheesey Egg Bagel ✔

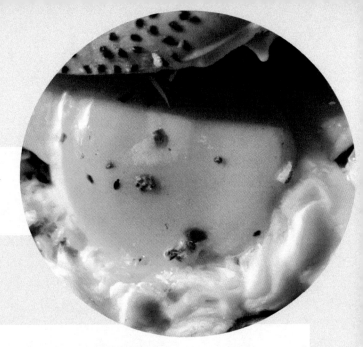

SERVINGS: 2 HALVES   PREPPING TIME: 5 MIN   COOKING TIME: 9-15 MIN

INGREDIENTS

- 1 bagel of choice, halved (I used The Better Bagel)
- 2 eggs
- 1/4 cup shredded low fat cheese (mozzarella or the three-cheese blend from Trader Joe's!)
- Red pepper flakes
- 1 tsp butter, melted
- salt and pepper to taste

DIRECTIONS

1. Preheat oven to 375F and line a baking sheet with parchment paper. It using an airfryer, line the airfryer!
2. Cut the bagel in half and brush the cut side with melted butter
3. Place the bagels cut side down and press them firmly into the parchment paper. This is important so the eggs don't leak.
4. Crack an egg into each bagel hole and season with salt and pepper.
5. Top with 1/4 cup shredded cheese
6. For runny yolks, bake for 10-12 minutes or airfry for 9 minutes at 350F. Increase time by 3 minutes for firmer yolks.

- ROYO Low Carb, HIGH FIBER Bread - [1 slice - 30 cal,, 11g Fiber] CODE: PROTEINSNACKQUEEN
- ROYO Low Carb Everything Bagel - [1 bagel- 80 cal] CODE: PROTEINSNACKQUEEN
- Gluten Free PAGEL 250 calories - 4g protein, 43g carbs, 8g fat
- The Better Bagel - 160 calories, 26g protein, 40g carbs, 2g fat
- Zero Carb Bagel - 90 calories, 14g protein, 14g carbs, 4 g fat

Calories for 1/2 a bagel: 258 | Carbohydrate: 21g | Protein: 23g | Fat: 10g

Chocolate Banana Chia Pudding ✅

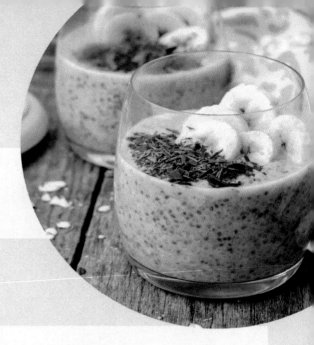

SERVINGS: 1	PREPPING TIME: 5 MIN	COOKING TIME: 0 MIN

INGREDIENTS

- 1 scoop of your favorite chocolate protein powder.
- 1/2 cup 0% Greek Yogurt
- 1.5 T chia seeds
- 1/4 ripe banana, sliced
- 1/4 cup unsweetened almond milk
- 1 tsp stevia drops or your favorite 0 calorie sweetener
- Optional: Add 1T of Cacao for extra chocolate flavor.

DIRECTIONS

1. Stir protein powder, yogurt, sweetener and chia seeds with milk.
2. Place banana sliced on top!
3. Place in the fridge overnight or for a couple of hours to set!

Tips:
- You can sub chocolate with any flavor to switch it up! I love Banana Cream!
- You can also omit protein powder alltogether, as this recipe will still be high in protein!

Calories: 294, Carbohydrate: 21g, Protein: 37g | Fat: 7g

Strawberry Chia Pudding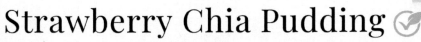

| SERVINGS: 1 | PREPPING TIME: 5 MIN | COOKING TIME: 0 MIN |

INGREDIENTS

- 1.5 T Chia seeds
- 1 Scoop Vanilla Protein Powder
- 1 tsp vanilla
- 2 tsp honey
- 1/4 cup 0% fat free greek yogurt
- 1/2 cup unsweetened plant milk (I'm using Almond Breeze)
- 2 T sugar free strawberry jam (I'm using Good Good)
- 3 strawberries, sliced

DIRECTIONS

1. Mix plant milk, vanilla, and protein powder with 1 T strawberry jam and 1 tsp honey.
2. Add chia seeds to the mixture and stir generously.
3. Place in the fridge for 15-20 min to set.
4. Mix Greek yogurt, 1 tsp honey, and 1 T Jam
5. Pour Greek yogurt mixture on top.
6. Chop 3 strawberries for garnish.

Calories: 295, Carbohydrate: 30g, Protein: 28g | Fat: 7 grams

Strawberry Vanilla Yogurt Toast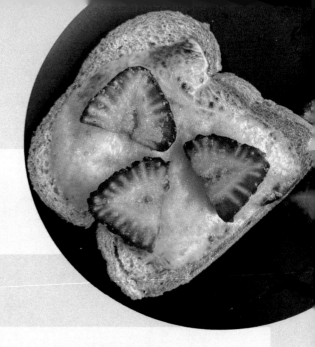

SERVINGS: 1   PREPPING TIME: 5 MIN   COOKING TIME: 7 MIN

INGREDIENTS

- ½ serving Vanilla Protein powder (Naked Whey)
- 1 slice low carb bread (Carbonaught bread or Royo Bread)
- 2 T Greek yogurt - fat free
- 1 T Good Good Strawberry Preserves
- 3 Strawberries, sliced thin
- 1 T liquid eggwhites
- 2 tsp Lakanto Golden Monkfruit Sweetener

DIRECTIONS

1. Stir protein powder into yogurt until combined
2. Mix in fruit preserve & liquid eggwhites,
3. Spread onto bread
4. Airfry bread for 7 min at 380F. You can also bake in a convection oven
5. Sprinkle monkfruit or alternative sugar of choice on top along with strawberry slices.

Calories: 160, Carbohydrate: 21g, Protein: 18g | Fat: 0grams

High-Protein Carrot Cake Overnight Oats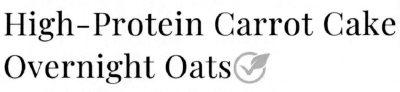

SERVINGS: 1	PREPPING TIME: 5 MIN	COOKING TIME: 0 MIN

INGREDIENTS

- 1/2 packet of Quaker Maple Brown Sugar Oatmeal Packet (may use Trader Joe's Maple Oatmeal)
- 2 scoops (30g) vanilla protein powder
- 2/3 cup (160g) unsweetened almond milk (or milk of choice)
- 1/4 c grated fresh carrots
- 10g golden raisins
- 5g crushed walnuts
- 1/4 tsp (1g) cinnamon
- 2 T Sugar Free Maple Syrup (Lakanto brand is the best)

DIRECTIONS

1. Stir together oats, protein powder, almond milk, carrots, raisins, walnuts, maple syrup and cinnamon.
2. Refrigerate oat mixture in mason jar or small container overnight.
3. Enjoy the next day!

Calories: 330, Carbohydrate: 37g, Protein: 28g | Fat: 7g

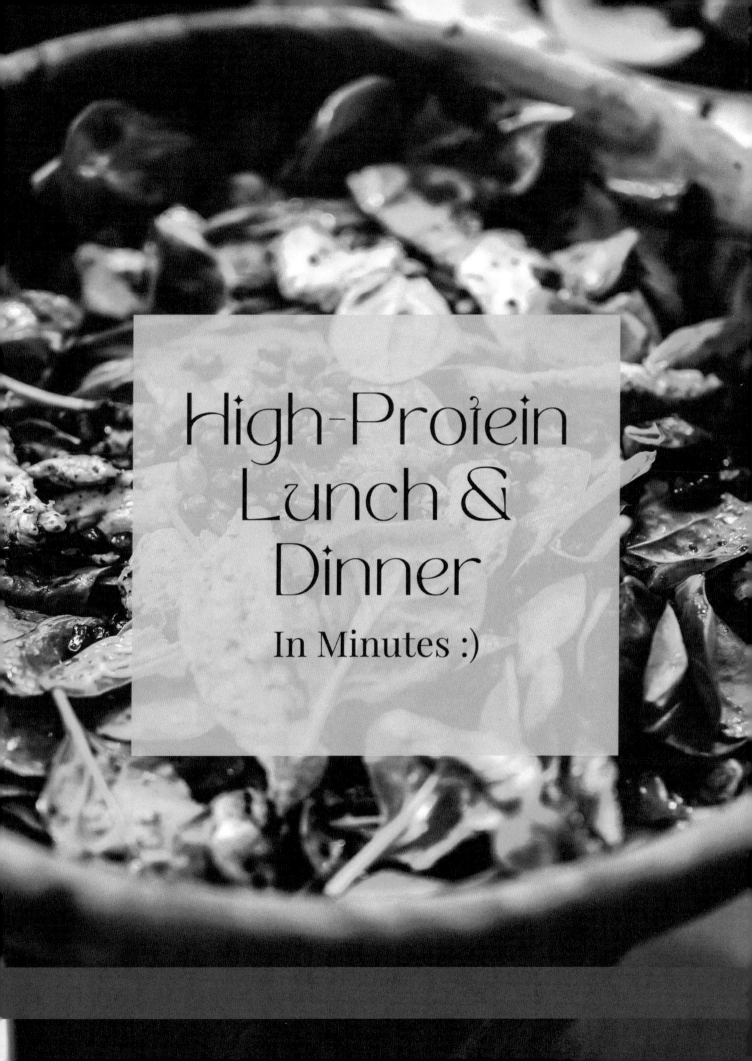

High-Protein Lunch & Dinner

In Minutes :)

High-Protein Chicken Salad [Wrap & Sandwich]

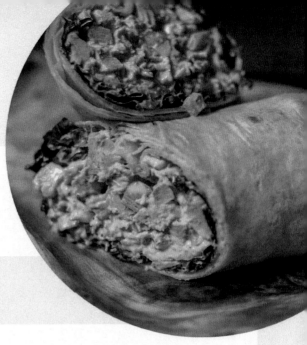

SERVINGS: 1	PREPPING TIME: 5 MIN	COOKING TIME: 0 MIN

INGREDIENTS

- 3.5 oz chicken breast, shredded
- 1/4 cup 0% Greek Yogurt (or Kitehill Greek Style Yogurt)
- 1/8 small red onion, diced
- 1 T Lite Mayo
- 1oz/1/4 cup of chopped red grapes
- 1.5 oz / 1/3 cup sliced celery
- 1/2 T Dijon mustard
- Ranch Powder (Trader Joes or
- Mission High Protein Tortilla Wrap, or Hero Bread High Protein Tortilla Wrap
- Royo or Equii Bread to make a Sandwich

DIRECTIONS

1. Placed 3.5 oz shredded chicken into a bowl
2. Mix together chicken, yogurt, dijon, mayonnaise, red onion, celery, grapes, Ranch powder, salt, and pepper.
3. If you're creating a wrap, spoon the mixture into wrap and wrap in preferred way.

10% off with code PROTEINSNACKQUEEN

Calories without Wrap: 190-205, Carbohydrate: 8 grams, Protein: 28 grams, Fat: 5 grams
Calories with Wrap: 311, Carbohydrate: 23 grams, Protein: 36 grams, Fat: 8 grams
Calories for Sandwich : 330 Carbohydrate: 32 grams, Protein: 34 grams, Fat: 8 grams

Easy Turkey Wrap (BLT Option included)

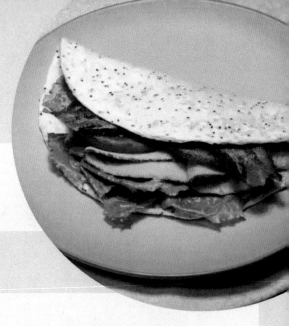

SERVINGS: 1   PREPPING TIME: 5 MIN   COOKING TIME: 0 MIN

INGREDIENTS

- 2 Egglife wraps or 1 high-protein wrap of choice (Mission High Protein Tortilla Wrap, or Hero Bread High Protein Tortilla)
- 2 T Lite Mayo
- 4 Slices of Smoked Turkey Breast
- 1 Slice of lite Cheddar
- 1 pickle spear, sliced in half
- 1 leaf of romaine lettuce

Optional to make BLT:

- 1 tomato, thinly sliced
- 2 slices of turkey bacon

DIRECTIONS

1. Warm 2 wraps in the microwave for 15 seconds (or on a stove if using wheat-based wrap).
2. Spread 1 T of lite mayo on each.
3. Place 2 slices of Smoked Turkey on each.
4. Place 1/2 slice of cheese on each.
5. Place 1/2 slice of pickle on each.
6. Place 1/2 romaine leaf on each.
7. If creating BLT version:
   a. Add 1-2 thin slices of tomato to each wrap followed by 1 slice of turkey bacon
8. Fold wraps in half and enjoy!

Calories with Egglife Wrap: 2 wraps: Calories: 297, Carbohydrate: 3 grams, Protein: 42 grams, Fat: 13 grams --- with Turkey Bacon: Calories: 335, Carbohydrate: 3 grams, Protein: 48 grams, Fat: 15 grams

Calories with Mission Wrap: 1 wrap: Calories: 280, Carbohydrate: 17 grams, Protein: 27 grams, Fat: 12 grams --- with Turkey Bacon: Calories: 317, Carbohydrate: 17 grams, Protein: 33 grams, Fat: 13 grams

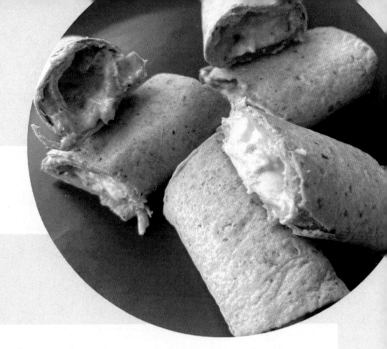

Cheesey Chicken Taquito

SERVINGS: 2 TAQUITOS   PREPPING TIME: 5 MIN   COOKING TIME:8 MIN

INGREDIENTS

- 2 high protein tortillas
- 2 oz shredded chicken breast
- 1/8 cup low fat cottage cheese
- 1.5 oz light shredded cheese (1/4 c + 1/8 cup)

DIRECTIONS

1. Mix chicken, cheese, & cottage cheese together.
2. Warm 2 tortillas and lay them flat.
3. Spoon half the mixture inton each tortilla.
4. Roll each tortilla tightly and fold the bottom.
5. Airfry at 380F for 7-8 minutes or until tortilla is crispy
6. Slice each tortilla in half and enjoy!

Calories: 230 | Carbohydrate: 18g | Protein: 23 g | Fat: 7 g

Lazy Chicken Caesar Wrap

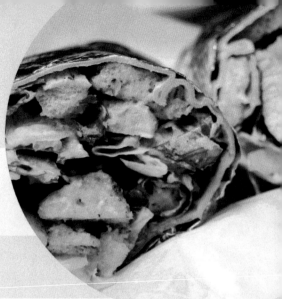

SERVINGS: 1   PREPPING TIME: 5 MIN   COOKING TIME: 0 MIN

INGREDIENTS

- 1 Folios Parmesan Cheese Wrap
- 2.5 oz Rotisserie Chicken Breast
- 3 T Bolthouse Farms Creamy Caesar
- Chopped Romaine
- Optional: Croutons

DIRECTIONS

1. Let wrap sit out for 5 minutes
2. Mix chicken with dressing
3. Chop lettuce
4. Wrap ingredient and season with salt and pepper

Calories: 324 | Carbohydrate: 6g | Protein: 32g | Fat: 19g

Lazy Buffalo Chicken Wrap

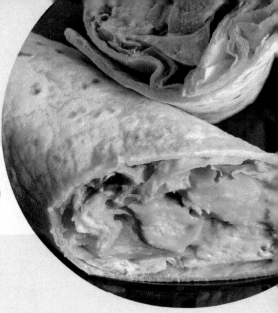

SERVINGS: 1   PREPPING TIME: 5 MIN   COOKING TIME: 0 MIN

INGREDIENTS

- 1 high-protein <u>Plant Powered Mission Tortilla</u>
- 4 T Buffalo Sauce
- 3 oz rotisserie chicken breast
- 3 T <u>Bolthouse Farms Classic Ranch</u>
- 1/4 cup light shredded 3 cheese Blend

DIRECTIONS

1. Heat wrap in microwave or on a stove top
2. Mix chicken with buffalo, ranch, and cheese.
3. Chop lettuce & build onto wrap.
4. Wrap tightly and enjoy!

Calories: 312, Carbohydrate: 21g, Protein: 32g | Fat: 11 grams

7-minute Spinach Dip Chicken Burger Sandwich

SERVINGS: 1   PREPPING TIME: 4 MIN   COOKING TIME: 3 MIN

INGREDIENTS

- 2 slices High Fiber Bread (Royo (code PROTEINSNACKQUEEN or Equii or Carb Savvy)
- 1 Amylu Kale & Mozzarella Chicken Burger or any Chicken Sausage of Choice - I like Bilinski's.
- 2 T Trader Joe's Spinach & Kale Greek Yogurt Dip
  - (Alternative: Good & Gather Spinach & Artichoke dip from Target)

DIRECTIONS

1. Toast your bread
2. Warm the chicken burger
3. Smear dip on one slice of bread
4. Break up chicken burger into pieces and layer on top of dip
5. Cover with 2nd slice of bread and enjoy!

Calories: 326, Carbohydrate: 31g, Protein: 28g | Fat: 10 grams

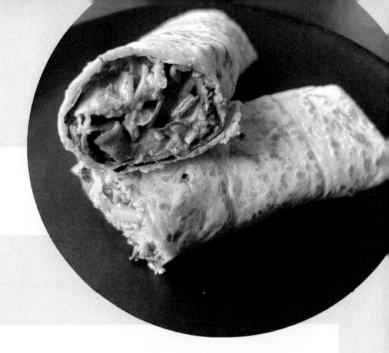

Southwest Style Chicken Wrap

SERVINGS: 1- 2   PREPPING TIME: 10 MIN   COOKING TIME: 0

INGREDIENTS

- 3 oz shredded chcicken breast - use rotisserie chicken for faster prep.
- 1/4 cup lite/ low fat shredded cheese
- 1/8 cup canned corn
- 1/8 cup of black beans
- 2 T fresh pico de gallo salsa
- A handful of chopped cilantro

Sauce:

- 1/4 cup 0%fat greek yogurt
- 1 T light mayonaise
- 1 T Taco Seasoning
- Juice of a 1/4 lime
- Dash of Siracha

DIRECTIONS

1. Mix chicken, cheese, beans, corn, salsa, and cilantro in a bowl
2. In a separate bowl mix yogurt, mayo, taco seasoning, lime, and siracha
3. Combine all ingredients and mix thoroughly until all ingredients are coated with sauce.
4. Heat up both tortillas on a skillet
5. Place half of mixture in each tortilla and roll tightly, closing off the edges by tucking them.
6. Place rolled tortillas on skillet to warm and secure shape.

Calories: 275 | Carbohydrate: 23g | Protein: 24 g | Fat: 10 g

Turkey Pinwheels

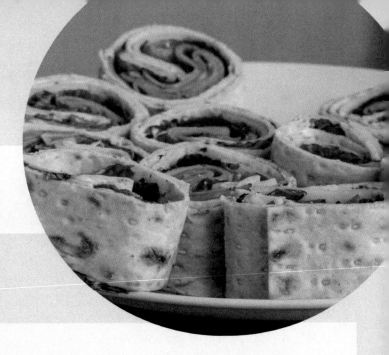

SERVINGS:2   PREPPING TIME: 10 MIN   COOKING TIME: 0

INGREDIENTS

- 1 Mission or Hero Tortilla
- 3 slices Smoked Turkey Breast
- 1 slice light cheddar cheese
- 4 T Spinach and Spinach & Kale Greek Yogurt Dressing
- 2 T Bolthouse Farms Italian Vinaigrette
- 1-2 leaves of romaine or iceberg lettuce

DIRECTIONS

1. Warm your tortilla then lay it flat.
2. Add smoked turkey slices & cheddar.
3. Smear 4 T Spinach and Kale Greek Yogurt Dip.
4. Drizzle 2 T of Bolthous Farms dressing.
5. Roll the tortilla tightly. You may use aluminum foil to ensure everything stays together.
6. Place in the fridge for 20 minutes
7. Cut into 4-5 wheels if you'd like.

Calories: 95 | Carbohydrate: 8g | Protein: 9 g | Fat: 3 g

Taco Pinwheels

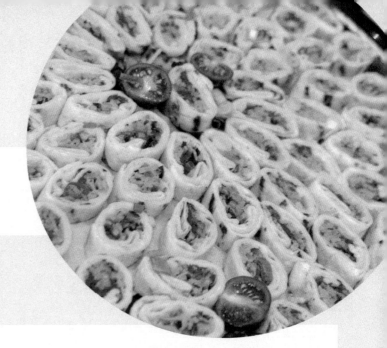

SERVINGS:15 BITES   PREPPING TIME: 10 MIN   COOKING TIME: 0 MIN
UNLESS COOKING CHICKEN

INGREDIENTS

- 4 oz shredded rotisserie chicken or Trader Joe's Pollo Asado
- 1-2 T Mild taco seasoning
- 1/3 cup lite Mexican Blend Cheese
- 2.5 oz reduced fat cream cheese
- 1/4 cup chopped bell peppers
- Chopped romaine
- 2 high protein tortillas

Optional dipping: Guacamole, salsa

DIRECTIONS

1. Bake/air fry your chicken and then shred it.
2. In a bowl, mix your chicken, taco seasoning, and cream cheese.
3. Add cheese and chopped bell peppers and chopped romaine
4. Lay two warm tortillas flat.
5. Spoon filling into each tortill.
6. Roll the tortilla tightly like a burrito
7. Place in the fridge for 20 min
8. Slice the tortilla into 7 pieces!

Calories: 54 | Carbohydrate: 5g | Protein: 3-4 g | Fat: 2 g

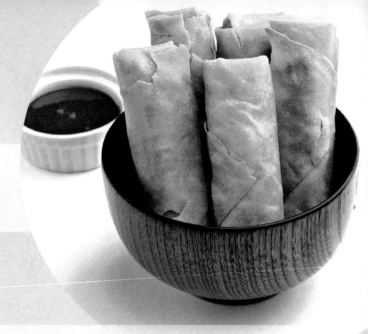

Cheeseburger Eggrolls

SERVINGS:1   PREPPING TIME: 5 MIN   COOKING TIME: 7 MIN OR 17 MIN
                                                   TO INCLUDE COOKING BEEF

INGREDIENTS

- 1 1/2 oz of lean ground beef (96%) (1/4 cup), cooked
- 1/8 cup light shredded cheese
- A pinch of chopped red onion
- 1 tablespoon of ketchup
- 1/2 T of light mayo
- A squirt of mustard
- Salt and pepper to taste
- A pickle, Julienned

DIRECTIONS

1. Cook lean ground beef - 96% is the leanest and lowest in calories but use whatever you'd like.
2. In a small bowl mix cooked ground beef, red onion, ketchup, mustard, mayo, salt, pepper, and cheese.
3. Once the mixture is coated, place in the middle of an eggroll wrapper.
4. Wet the edges of the egg roll, wrapper and fold in like a burrito. The wet edges should stick together.
5. Place an egg roll in air fryer and air fry at 380° for 7 minutes or until crispy.

Calories for per egg roll: 190 | Carbohydrate: 20g | Protein: 31 g | Fat: 6g

10-minute Pizza Roll Ups

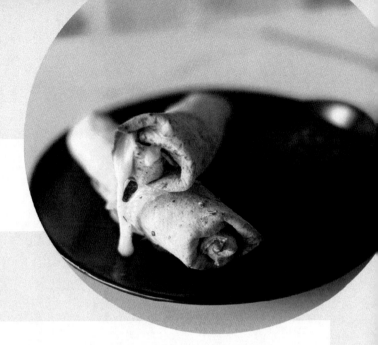

SERVINGS: 1 ROLL UP   PREPPING TIME: 5 MIN   COOKING TIME: 7 MIN

INGREDIENTS

- 1 protein wrap (I used <u>Mission Plant Powered Protein Tortilla in the Garlic Herb Flavor</u>
- 1/2 T pizza sauce
- Reduced fat mozzarella cheese stick, sliced in half the long way
- 4 Turkey Pepperonis, sliced in quarters - I used Applegate.
- 1/8 cup lite cheese blend (add cottage cheese for extra protein)
- Italian Seasoning Blend

Optional Topper:
- 1/2 tsp melted garlic
- Italian Seasoning Blend
- Parmesan Cheese

DIRECTIONS

1. Lay a tortilla on a flat surface
2. Spoon 1/2 tablespoon of pizza sauce on tortilla and spread toward the edges, ensuring the sauce isn't too thick anywhere. Leave edges dry
3. Slice a mozzarella stick in half vertically (the long way)
4. Slice 4 turkey pepperonis into quarters
5. Lay one half of a mozz stick down, then the other half about an inch away. Spread turkey slices in between
6. Spread 1/8 cup of shredded cheese of choice into mixture.
7. Fold the edges in first, then begin rolling the tortilla away from you, making sure there are no holes on the sides.
8. Airfry at 400F for 7 minutes of bake at 400F for 10 minutes!

Calories per serving: 233 | Carbohydrate: 16g | Protein: 22g | Fat: 9g

Easiest 5-Minute Cheese Quesadillas

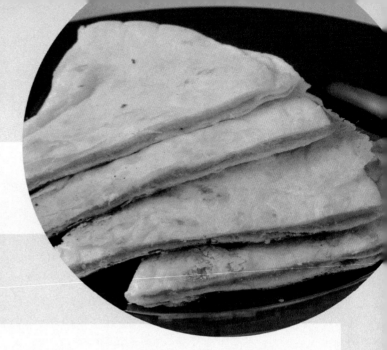

SERVINGS: 2   PREPPING TIME: 0 MIN   COOKING TIME: 5 MIN

INGREDIENTS

- 2 Carb Savvy Tortilla from Trader Joes or <u>Carb Friendly Tortillas</u>
- 1/2 cup shredded fat free or Lite Mexican Blend. If you use fat free, rinse the cheese first so it melts easier!

(You can add ground meat if you have that on hand and any other fillings like chopped veggies! I like to keep this one simple :))

- Optional Additional Ingredients:
  - Fresh Salsa, Guacamole,

DIRECTIONS

1. Heat a pan and spray a light coating of cooking spray. You can also use the extra fast method and heat the tortilla directly on a stove flame for charr.
2. Once the tortilla is warm, sprinkle cheese on one half of the tortilla.
3. Place a lid over the pan to melt the cheese.
4. Once the cheese is slightly melted, feel free to add additional ingredients. Then fold tortilla in half.
5. With a spatula, press the tortilla flat and cook

Calories per quesadilla: 138 | Carbohydrate: 11g | Protein: 11g | Fat: 6g

BBQ Chicken Jicama Tacos

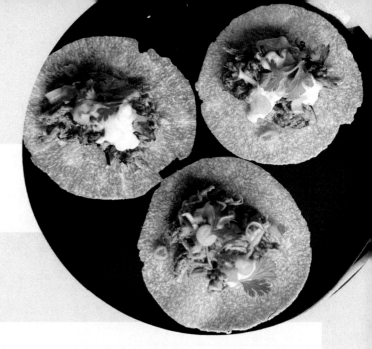

SERVINGS:1   PREPPING TIME: 5 MIN   COOKING TIME: 5 MIN. IF MAKING CHICKEN, 25 MIN TOTAL

INGREDIENTS

- 4 jicama tacos from Trader Joe's or thinly sliced jicama OR butter lettuce

Filling:

- 4 oz chicken breast from rotisserie chicken, or cooked chicken breast
- 1/4 cup red onions
- 1 oz/ 1/4 cup low fat shredded mozzarella cheese
- 6 T bbq sauce- I used reduced calorie, no sugar added Primal Kitchen Foods

Topping:

- A quarter green onion, chopped
- A bunch of cilantro, de-stemmed
- Bolthouse Farms Ranch as a drizzle

DIRECTIONS

- 1. Chop red onion and shred chicken breast!
- 2. Mix filling ingredients until all chicken is coated.
- 3. Spray an air fryer tray with avocado oil
- 4. Place filling in air fryer and Airfry for 5 min at 380F.
- 5. Chop green onion and de Stem cilantro 6. Lay out jicama taco on a plate. Add 1.5-2oz cooked mixture in the center of each taco!
- 7. Drizzle with green onion, cilantro and ranch and ENJOY!

Calories for 4 tacos: 258 | Carbohydrate: 20g | Protein: 31 g | Fat: 6g

Ashley's Favorite Salmon Wrap

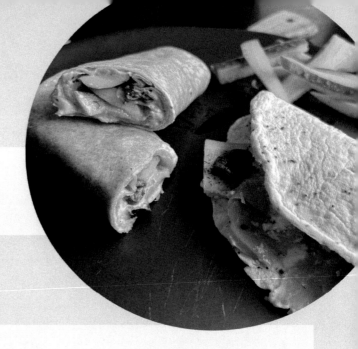

SERVINGS: 1   PREPPING TIME: 5 MIN   COOKING TIME: 0

INGREDIENTS

- 1 lavash tortilla or Egglife Everything but the Bagel Wrap, or a any protein tortilla of your choice!
- 1 T light cream cheese
- 2 T fat free or low fat cottage cheese
- A Persian cucumber sliced flat and thin
- 2 oz Smoked Salmon (I'm using Everything but the bagel Salmon from Trader Joe's)
- Everything but the Bagel Seasoning
- Dill Pickle seasoning
- 2-3 olives or 1 T Kalamata olives, sliced
- 1/2 lemon juice

DIRECTIONS

1. In a small bowl, mix cottage cheese and cream cheese with seasonings and lemon and blend to whip.
2. Peel and slice your cucumber thin and flat.
3. Warm your tortilla or lay out your Egglife wrap flat.
4. Smear cheese blend into wrap
5. Add salmon cucumbers and olives. Season more.
6. Wrap or fold to enjoy!

Calories for Lavash Wrap Version: 260 | Carbohydrate: 17g | Protein: 35 g | Fat: 11 g
Calories for Egglife Wrap Version: 200 | Carbohydrate: 6g | Protein: 34 g | Fat: 9 g

Cottage Cheese
Bruschetta Toast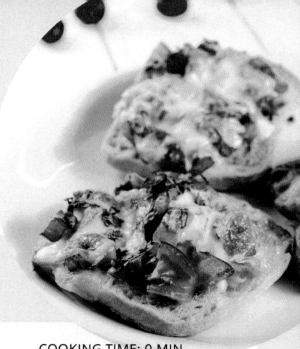

SERVINGS: 1	PREPPING TIME: 5 MIN	COOKING TIME: 0 MIN

INGREDIENTS

- 2 pieces of toast, I love ROYO
- 2 T Store Bought Bruschetta or chopped tomatoes & basil
- 3/4 cup fat free or low fat cottage cheese

DIRECTIONS

1. Toast 2 slices of low carb bread
2. Blend with an immersion blender or coffee frother 3/4 cup of fat-free cottage cheese.
3. Scoop half of the whipped cottage cheese on each piece of toast
4. Top with 1 T of bruschetta each.
5. Sprinkle with salt and pepper and enjoy!

Fat free cottage cheese, 2 slices of Royo Bread & 2 T Trader Joe's Bruschetta
Calories: 270 | Carbohydrate: 33g | Protein: 26g | Fat:3g

Greek-Inspired Chicken Hummus Wrap

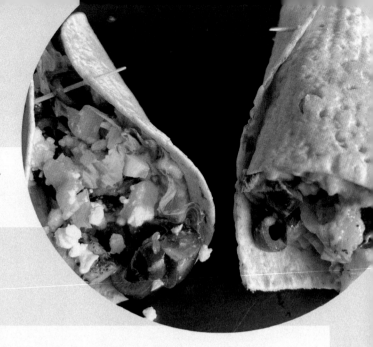

SERVINGS:1   PREPPING TIME: 10 MIN   COOKING TIME: 0 MIN OR 20 MIN IF COOKING CHICKEN

INGREDIENTS

- 1 Carb Savvy tortilla OR 1/2 lavash bread
- 1.5 oz cooked chicken breast, sliced
- 1 T Kalamata Olives (7g)
- 1/4 cup fat free feta cheese
- 2 T spicy hummus dip (50 cal per serving)
- 2 T low fat Italian dressing (Bolthouse Farms, Skinny Girl are both great options)
- 1/2 a Persian cucumber, Juliened

DIRECTIONS

1. Use pre-cooked chicken for this otherwise bake/airfry your chicken at 380F for 15-18 min! Season prior to baking: I used the 21 seasoning salute from Trader Joe's!
2. Once finished, mix dressing with chicken in a small bowl
3. Lay out tortilla on a flat surface and smear hummus in the middle
4. Add chicken
5. Julienne a Persian cucumber and lay flat next to chicken
6. Add chopped tomato, feta, olives and lettuce & enjoy!

Calories per serving for Carb Savvy Tortilla: 250 | Carbohydrate: 22g | **Protein: 24g** | Fat: 8g

Calories per serving for Lavash Bread: 213 | Carbohydrate: 18g | **Protein: 21g** | Fat: 6g

Cheeseburger Quesadillas

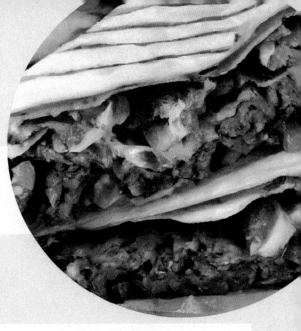

SERVINGS: 1   PREPPING TIME: 5 MIN   COOKING TIME: 5 MIN

INGREDIENTS

- 1 high protein tortilla (I love Hero, but Mission works too!)
- 3.5 oz 93-96 ground lean beef (Trader Joe's carries 96 lean)
- 1 oz Fat free or low fat cheese
- 1 T red onion, chopped
- 1 T ketchup
- 1 T lite mayo
- 1/2 tsp mustard
- 1 chopped pickle
- 1 Romaine lettuce

DIRECTIONS

1. Place 3.5 oz ground beef on a tortilla.
2. Toss a sprinkle of chopped onion on top.
3. Grease a skillet on medium heat and turn the tortilla BEEF-SIDE down. Let it cook for 3-5 minutes.
4. Once cooked, flip tortilla over so beef side is up. Add cheese and cover the skillet so the cheese melts.
5. Remove from heat, add ketchup, mustard, mayo & chopped pickle and chopped romaine.
6. Fold in half and slice down the middle!

Calories for 96/4 beef : 370 Carbohydrate: 24g Protein: 38g, Fat: 15g

Trader Joe's Gyro Sandwich

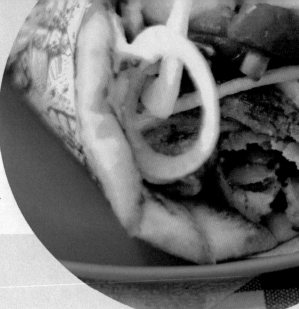

SERVINGS: 1   PREPPING TIME: 10 MIN   COOKING TIME:

INGREDIENTS

- 1 High Protein Tortilla - I used Mission
- 2 oz Greek Gyro Meat from Trader Joe's
- 3 T Trader Joe's Cucumber Tzatziki Dip
- 1/4 cup Fat Free Feta Cheese
- 1 few slices of onion
- 2-3 slices of tomato

DIRECTIONS

1. Not Pictured in the video, but warm your meat on a skillet or in the air fryer (3 min at 380F) for more flavor.
2. Warm your preferred tortilla on a flame, skillet or in the microwave
3. Chop a few slices of tomato and onion.
4. Lay the meat in the tortilla, add 2 Tzatziki dip, feta, and tomato and onion.
5. Fold wrap in half and enjoy!

Calories: 375 | Carbohydrate: 26g | Protein: 30g | Fat: 17g

Greek Cottage Cheese Bowl ✅

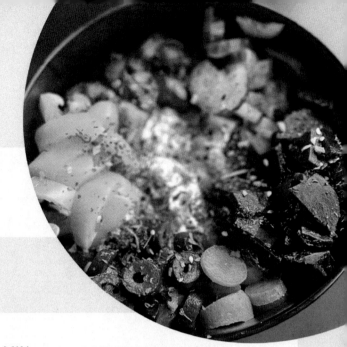

SERVINGS: 1   **PREPPING TIME: 10 MIN**   **COOKING TIME: 0 MIN**

INGREDIENTS

- 1 cup (280g) 0% cottage cheese (Trader Joe's) or low-fat cottage cheese
- 1-2 tbsp (20g) kalamata olives, sliced
- 1/2 c sliced Persian cucumber, sliced
- 5-10 halved cherry tomatoes
- 1-2 mini peppers, sliced
- 1-2 baby carrots, sliced
- 1/2 cup boiled beets (optional)
- 2 T Trader Joe's Cucumber Tzatziki dip or ANY Tzatziki Dip
- 1/2 tsp (0.5g) dill and/or chives (optional)
- Everything But the Bagel Seasoning

DIRECTIONS

1. Top cottage cheese with ingredients and ENJOY!

Calories: 255 | Carbohydrate: 17g | Protein: 32g | Fat: 7g

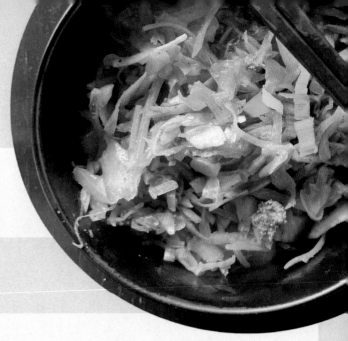

Spring Roll in a Bowl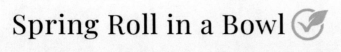

SERVINGS: 4   PREPPING TIME: 5 MIN   COOKING TIME: 10 MIN

INGREDIENTS

- 1 lb 96/4 lean ground beef (or tofu)
- 1.5 bags shredded cabbage
- 1 cup shredded carrots
- 2 green onions, chopped
- 1/4 yellow onion chopped
- 1 T sesame oil
- 2 cloves garlic, minced or 1/2 T minced
- 1 tsp ginger
- 1/4 c coconut aminos
- Garlic power
- Salt & Pepper

DIRECTIONS

1. Heat a skillet with sesame oil.
2. Cook chopped yellow onion, garlic and beef
3. Add cabbage, carrot, green onion, ginger, coconut aminos, and seasoning
4. Cook for 5 minutes until all ingredients are cooked through
5. Season with garlic powder, crushed red pepper, salt and pepper!

Make this lower calorie by replacing beef with lean ground chicken or turkey

Calories per serving: 230 | Carbohydrate: 16g | Protein: 24g | Fat: 8g

Ashley's Egg Salad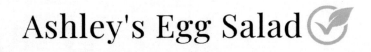

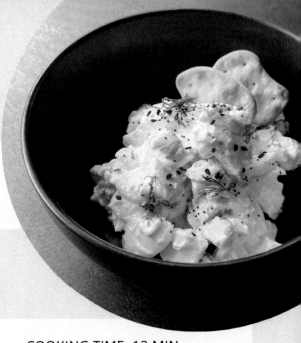

SERVINGS: 1   PREPPING TIME: 8 MIN   COOKING TIME: 12 MIN
                                                    (FOR HARD BOILED EGGS)

INGREDIENTS

- 2 whole eggs, hard boiled and chopped
- 2 egg whites, hard boiled and chopped
- 1 T Fat Free Greek Yogurt
- 1/2 T Lite Hellman's Mayo
- 1/2 tsp Dijon Mustard
- 1 T chopped green onions
- 1 T Dill
- Everything But the Bagel Seasoning

Optional: Bread/wrap

DIRECTIONS

1. Mix together eggs, egg whites, Greek yogurt, Lite Mayo, Dijon & Everything but the bagel seasoning
2. Add chopped green onion & dill & stir more
3. Enjoy

Calories: 219, Carbohydrate: 4g | Protein: 24g | Fat: 12g

Cheeseburger Bowl

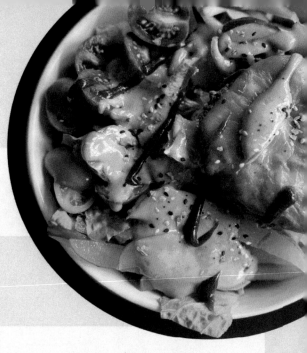

SERVINGS: 1   PREPPING TIME: 10 MIN   COOKING TIME: 7 MIN

INGREDIENTS

- 5 oz ground lean beef OR Roast Beef Deli Meat for QUICK version
- 2-3 leaves romaine, chopped
- 1 oz/ slice Fat free or low fat cheese of choice
- 1 small tomato, chopped
- 1/4 cup chopped red onion
- 1 dill pickle, chopped
- Paprika, garlic powder
- Salt and pepper to taste

Sauce:
- 2 T Lite Mayo
- 2 T Ketchup
- 1/2 Tsp Mustard

DIRECTIONS

1. If you want to make patties, mix beef and an egg along with seasoning in a bowl and mold into patties. You will just be breaking this up anyway so may be easier to just use ground beef.
2. Cook the beef and season with paprika, garlic powder, salt and pepper. Add pickle juice for extra flavor. If you're using roast beef, place on a plate and top with cheese. Warm in the oven or microwave until the cheese melts.
3. Chop vegetables while the meat warms
4. Lay chopped lettuce in a bowl
5. Place 5 oz cooked meat on one side
6. Add remaining chopped ingredients
7. Mix Sauce ingredients together and drizzle on top!

Calories: 340 | Carbohydrate: 11 grams | Protein: 40 grams | Fat: 15 grams

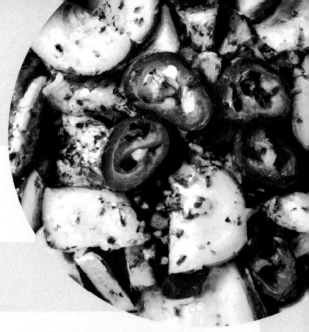

Cucumber Chili Crunch Salad

SERVINGS: 1   PREPPING TIME: 10 MIN   COOKING TIME: 0 MIN OR 20 MIN IF COOKING CHICKEN

INGREDIENTS

- 2 Persian cucumber, sliced
- 3-4 mini peppers, chopped
- 2 T Yai Thai Ginger Garlic Stirfry Sauce or your favorite low calorie ginger dressing
- 1 T Soy Sauce
- 3 oz chicken breast
- 1/2 T chili crunch, oil strained
- Everything But the Bagel Seasoning

DIRECTIONS

1. Pour soy sauce over chicken breast and cook/airfry
2. Chop cucumbers & peppers and toss into a bowl
3. Drizzle Ginger Garlic sauce on top.
4. Strain chili crunch oil and add chili crunch
5. Season with Everything But the Bagel seasoning.
6. Enjoy!

Calories: 240 | Carbohydrate: 15g | Protein: 30g | Fat: 7g

Feta & Cheddar Stuffed Mini Peppers

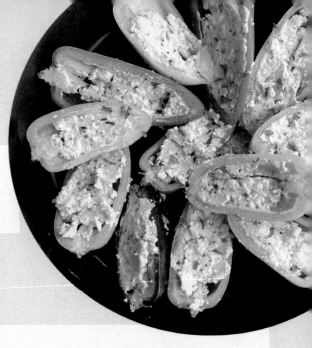

SERVINGS: 1 (12 PEPPERS)   PREPPING TIME: 10 MIN   COOKING TIME: 0 MIN

INGREDIENTS

- 1/2 lb mini peppers, sliced in half
- 1/4 cup fat free feta cheese
- 2 light laughing cow cheddar cheese wedges
- Everything But the Bagel Seasoning
- 1/2 tsp Chili Crunch, oil drained

DIRECTIONS

1. Slice mini peppers in half vertically to create a flat surface you can smear cheese on
2. Mix feta, cheddar, seasoning and chili crunch into a bowl.
3. Warm mixture in the microwave for 30 seconds to soften and to mix thoroughly.
4. Smear cheese paste onto each pepper!
5. Enjoy!

Calories per pepper: 12 | Carbohydrate: 2g | Protein: 1g | Fat: 0g

Hamburger-Meatloaf Bites

SERVINGS: 1   PREPPING TIME: 10 MIN   COOKING TIME: 20-30 MIN

INGREDIENTS

- 1 lb 96% lean ground beef
- 1/2 cup bread crumbs. PRO TIP: Use SnackHouse Keto Puffs (CODE PROTEINSNACKQUEEN for 15%) or Quest Chips
- 1/ cup shredded light cheddar cheese or cheese blend
- 1 cup eggwhites
- 1/4 ketchup
- 1/8 cup lite mayo
- 1/8 cup mustard
- 1/4 cup parmesan cheese
- Pickles/relish
- 1 T garlic powder
- 1 T onion powder

DIRECTIONS

1. Spray avocado oil on a pan & brown 1lb of lean ground beef.
2. Preheat oven to 400F.
3. Mix egg whites, cheese, 1 bag keto puffs/quest chips, or 1/2 cup breadcrumbs with 1/2 cup parmesan cheese, 1/4 cup ketchup, 1/8 cup light mayo, 1/8 cup mustard, pickles, garlic and onion powder.
4. Add cooked beef to the mixture and mix.
5. Grease 2 muffin trays (24 total) and fill each tray with mixture.
6. Bake in the oven for 20-30 minutes!
7. Serve with a side of ketup!

Calories per patty: 50, Carbohydrate: 1 gram, Protein: 6 grams, Fat: 2 grams

Korean-Inspired Vegetable Pancakes

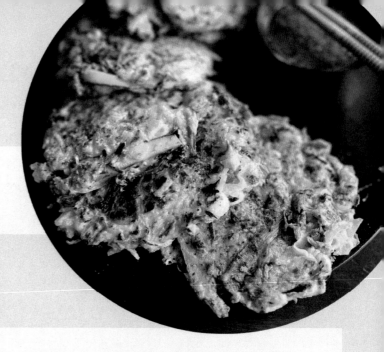

SERVINGS: 6 PATTIES   PREPPING TIME: 15 MIN   COOKING TIME: 10-15 MIN

INGREDIENTS

- 3/4 c all purpose flour
- 1/4 cup flavorless casein protein powder
- 1 t cornstartch
- 1 cup cold water
- 1/2 cup grated carrots
- 1/2 cup chopped cabbage
- 1cup grated leek greens
- 1/2 cup bean sprouts
- 1/4 yellow onion
- 3 green onion stalks chopped
- 1 cup cooked shrimp (150g)
- 1/2 cup sliced zucchini
- 1/2 -1 minced jalepano
- Optional: kelp noodles

Sauce:
- 2 T Trader Joe's Soyaki Sauce
- 1 T water

Alternative Dressing : 2 T soy sauce, 1 T sugar, 1/2 tsp
granulated garlic, 1 tspground ginger,1/2 tsp onion powder,
1/2 tsp sesame oil, 1/2 tsp sesame seeds

DIRECTIONS

1. Mix flour, protein, salt, and cornstartch with cold water, adding water slowly.
2. Add the rest of the ingredients and mix until all vegetables and shrimp are coated.
3. Heat a pan on high heat with oil.
4. Place a glob of batter and vegetables onto the skillet and let it simmer, turning down the heat to medium after initial sear
5. Cook each pancake until both sides are golden brown and crispy!
6. Mix dipping sauce and enjoy!

Calories per patty: 115 | Carbohydrate: 20g | Protein: 12 g | Fat: 1 g

Greek-Inspired Chicken Patties

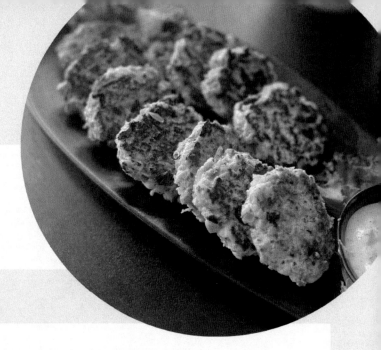

SERVINGS: 11 PATTIES   PREPPING TIME: 15 MIN   COOKING TIME: 15- 20 MIN

INGREDIENTS

- 20 oz raw ground chicken breast
- 60g fat free feta or 1/2 cup
- 1/4 cup Kalamata olives or 30g
- 1/4 cup greek yogurt (not included in video)
- 1/4 cup bread crumbs
- 1/4 onion
- 1/4 cup spinach
- 1-2 Eggs

GREEK SEASONING:

- 2 tsp oregano
- 2 tsp dried basil
- 1 tsp dried parsley
- 1 tsp onion powder
- 1 tsp garlic powder
- 1/2 tsp - thyme, rosemary
- Salt & pepper

DIRECTIONS

1. Use pre-marinated greek chicken if you can find it. Otherwise combine ALL ingredients into a bowl and mix. Try not to OVER-mix.
2. Form even-sized patties (should make about 11)
3. Oil a skillet and place each patty on skillet for about 3-5 minutes on medium heat until golden brown, then flip!
4. Cook second side until golden brown.
5. Remove from skillet and plate.
6. Dip in tzatziki sauce and enjoy!

1. Tzatziki option: Trader Joe's or Good Foods Tzatziki.
2. Bun option: ROYO Bread Burger Bun! (PROTEINSNACKQUEEN for 10% off)

Calories for each patty: 80 | Carbohydrate: 2g | Protein: 13g | Fat: 2g

Cobb Salad

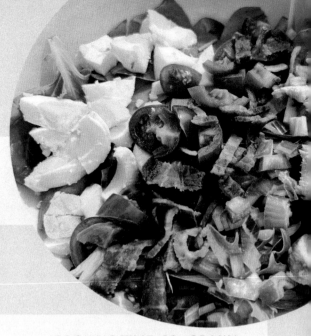

SERVINGS: 1   PREPPING TIME: 5 MIN   COOKING TIME: 20 - 25 MIN
(TIME TO COOK CHICKEN, BACON,
AND EGGS)

INGREDIENTS

- 2 cups (42g) mixed greens
- 1/2 chopped romaine heart
- 1 hard-boiled egg, quartered
- 1 slice of cooked turkey bacon, torn
- 4 oz (56g) cooked chicken breast, sliced or 4 slices Smoked Turkey Breast
- 1 handful cherry tomatoes, chopped
- 1 oz low-fat shredded cheese
- 1 handful of chopped mini pepper
- 1 persian cucumber
- 1/8 small red onion, sliced
- 1 chopped pickle
- 4 T Bolthouse Ranch Dressing
- Salt and pepper to taste

DIRECTIONS

1. Cook bacon and chicken/turkey if needed!
2. Chop egg, mini peppers, cucumber, onion, egg, romaine, & pickles!
3. Mix all ingredients together!
4. Pour dressing over salad, mix and enjoy!

Calories: 400 | Carbohydrate: 28g | Protein: 41 g | Fat: 14 g

45

Beet & Feta Salad

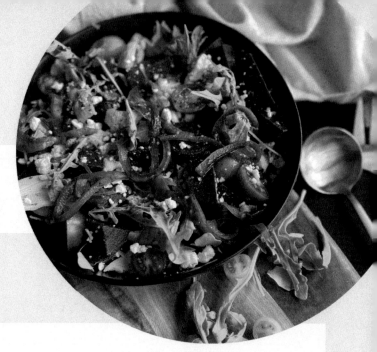

SERVINGS: 1   PREPPING TIME: 10 MIN   COOKING TIME: 0

INGREDIENTS

- 1 package of Trader Joe's Steamed Beets or 8 oz Cooked Beets
- 2 oz Fat Free Feta
- 1 package of Trader Joe's marinated Artichoke hearts
- 1 T pickled onions (optional but so good)
- 1 handful cherry tomatoes, chopped
- A bunch of arugula

Dressing:
- 1/2 T olive oil
- 1 T Balsamic Vinegar
- 1/4 tsp honey
- Salt & pepper

DIRECTIONS

1. Chop beets & tomatoes.
2. Sprinkle arugala in a bowl.
3. Add beets, tomatoes, feta, pickled onions, artichoke hearts.
4. In a small bowl, mix dressing ingredients. Drizzle on top of salad and mix.
5. Add salt and pepper to taste and enjoy!

Calories: 280 | Carbohydrate: 48g | Protein: 15 g | Fat: 7 g

Asian-Inspired
Kelp Noodle Salad

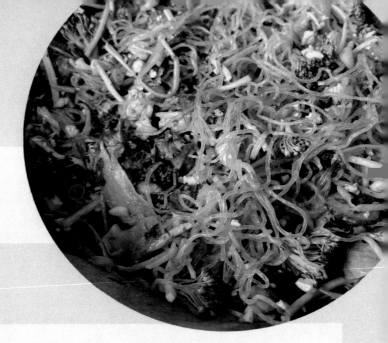

SERVINGS:2   PREPPING TIME: 10 MIN   COOKING TIME: 20 IF
                                                    COOKING CHICKEN

INGREDIENTS

- 7 oz chicken breast- seasoned with furikake and brushed with Soy sauce, cooked & chopped
- 12 oz shredded cabbage, broccoli, and carrot blend
- 1/2 heart of romaine, chopped
- 1/2 cup edamame beans
- A handful green onion, chopped
- 30g sushi ginger (Amazon or Whole Foods)
- Shredded toasted seaweed snacks
- 1/2 bag Kelp Noodles
- 1 Persian cucumber, chopped
- 1/4 cup chopped cilantro
- Furikake seasoning

Dressing:

- 3/4 c PB2 powder (45g)
- 1/4 c coconut aminos or soy sauce
- 1T rice wine vingegar
- 1 T grated ginger
- 1T honey
- 4T water
- 1/2 lime sprinkled on top

DIRECTIONS

1. Airfry or bake chicken.
2. Empty chopped cabbage, broccoli and carrot blend into a large bowl.
3. Add chopped romaine, edamame, green onion, cilantro, seaweed snacks, cucumber, and sushi ginger!
4. Wash and drain kelp noodles. Using only half the bag, begin to chop the noodles into shorter lengths. Toss into the bowl!
5. Combine ingredients to make dressing and pour over.
6. Season with furikake seasoning!

Calories: 350 | Carbohydrate: 36g | Protein: 40 g | Fat: 6 g

Crunchy Edamame Chicken Salad with Honey Sesame Dressing

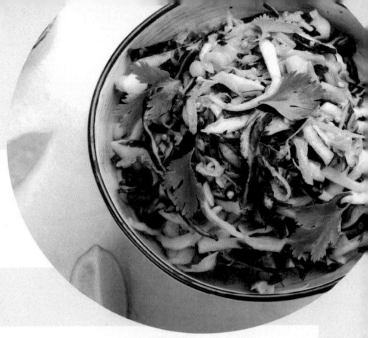

SERVINGS: 2   PREPPING TIME: 15 MIN   COOKING TIME: 20 IF COOKING CHICKEN

INGREDIENTS

- 4 oz edamame beans (soy beans)
- 1 bag chopped cabbage (or 1/2 a cabbage)
- 1/2 bag shredded carrots, or 3 shaved carrots
- 4 oz snap peas, cut into halves
- 3 radishes, sliced thin
- 3 green onions, chopped
- 3 sprigs mint, chopped
- Small bunch chopped cilantro
- 6 oz chicken

Dressing:
- 1/4 cup rice vinegar
- 1/4 cup coconut aminos
- 1 T Korean chili flakes
- 2 T sesame oil
- 2 T honey
- 1 T ginger, grated
- Furikake Seasoning

DIRECTIONS

1. Cut the snap peas and blanch them with the edamame beans for 2 minutes in salted water
2. Drain and chill
3. Marinate and cook chicken with 2 T coconut aminos, 2 T rice vinegar and 1/2 T sesame oil with salt and pepper.
4. Chop all remaining vegetables then add all vegetables to a bowl
5. Whisk dressing then add snap peas and edamame to salad.
6. Once chicken is done, add to the bowl!
7. Pour dressing right on top and serve immediately!

Calories: 350 | Carbohydrate: 36g | Protein: 40 g | Fat: 6 g

TABLE OF CONTENTS

Elote Salad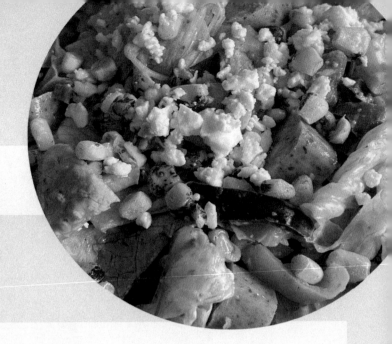

| SERVINGS: 1 | PREPPING TIME: 10 MIN | COOKING TIME: 10 MIN |

INGREDIENTS

- 1 cup corn (frozen fire roasted from Trader Joe's is great, but any works!)
- 1 cup Frozen Chopped Bell Peppers
- 1 chicken sausage, jalepeno flavor unless you prefer something milder
- 1/4 cup shredded parmesan cheese
- 1/4 cup crumbled fat free feta OR cojita cheese
- 1/2 jalepeno, seeded and chopped
- 1 green onion, chopped
- 1/4 cup red onion, chopped
- 1/2 bag chopped romaine lettuce or butter lettuce, or1 heart of romaine chopped
- 1.5 T Everything But the Elote Seasoning (or 1 tsp paprika, 1/4 tsp cumin, 1/4 tsp chile powder)
- Salt & Pepper to taste

Dressing:
- 1/4 cup T Cilantro Lime Vinagrette from Trader Joes
- Squeeze of 1/2 a Lime

OR From Scratch, blended:
- 1/4 cup lime juice
- 2 T Lite Mayonaise
- 1/2 cup cilantro
- 1/2 tsp Smoked Paprika
- Salt & Pepper

DIRECTIONS

1. Warm a medium sauce pan with a T of oil. Add corn and peppers and cook.
2. Once cooked, turn off heat to cool
3. Chop 1/4 red onion, green onion, jalapeño and add to the cooled pan of corn and peppers.
4. Add parmesan cheese, elote seasoning, salt, & pepper and stir.
5. Chop chicken sausage (warm or cold) and add to mixture.
6. In a separate bowl, combine salad mixture with chopped romaine . Pour 1/4 cup Cilantro Dressing and lime on top and stir!
7. Sprinkle with fat free feta cheese & enjoy!

If you prefer to eat this salad extra cold, refrain from including dressing until the very last step!

Calories per serving: 403 | Carbohydrate: 34g | Protein: 32 g | Fat: 16 g

Cucumber Ginger Sashimi Salad

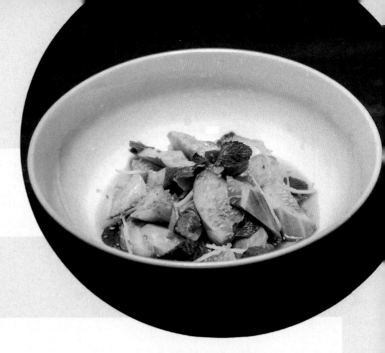

SERVINGS: 1   PREPPING TIME: 5 MIN   COOKING TIME: 0

INGREDIENTS

- 3 persian cucumbers, chopped
- Protein: 3 oz sashimi grade salmon or 4-5 oz Simply Surimi Crabstick, or pre-cooked shrimp
- 1/4 cup sushi ginger
- Furikake Seasoning

Dressing:

- 2 T Soy sauce
- 1 T Rice Wine Vinegar
- 1/2 tsp Toastest Sesame Oil

DIRECTIONS

1. Chop cucumbers into cubes or thin slices and place in a bowl
2. Cut protein to your liking and add
3. Add sushi ginger and furikake seasoning
4. In a separate bowl, mix soy sauce, rice wine vinegar, and toasted sesame oil.
5. Pour dressing over salad and ENJOY!

Quick Tip:
Replace Crab stick with Crab, Shrimp. Fish, Scallop, Crab Claws

Calories with Simply Surimi Crabstick:
250 | Carbohydrate: 36g | Protein: 19 g | Fat: 3 g

The Best High-Protein, Low-Carb Pasta Salad

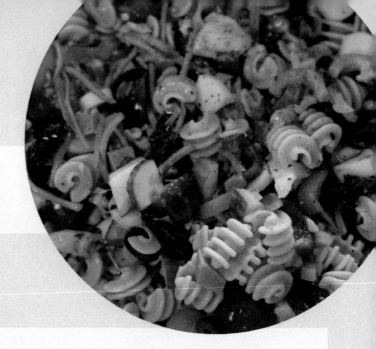

SERVINGS: 3	PREPPING TIME: 10 MIN	COOKING TIME: 10 MIN

INGREDIENTS

- 1/2 box Kaizen Pasta (250g)
- 2 light mozzarella sticks, chopped
- 10-15 cherry tomatoes, halved
- 5 persian cucumbers, chopped
- 1/4 red onion, finely chopped
- 5-6 sweet mini peppers or 1 bell pepper, chopped
- 1/4 (1 oz) cup kalamata olives
- 4 oz Trader Joe's Turkey Summer Sausage OR Applegate Turkey Pepperoni or ANY chicken sausage of choice, chopped
- 1 oz sundried tomatoes, oil-free & chopped
- 1 bag marinated artichoke hearts or 1/2 cup, chopped
- handful of chopped fresh parsley
- 1/4 cup Skinny Girl Italian Dressing or Bolthouse Farms Italian
- Salt & Pepper

DIRECTIONS

1. Cook the pasta according to the box instructions
2. Chop all ingredients while pasta cooks
3. Drain pasta and add to a large bowl
4. Add all chopped ingredients, salt, pepper, and dressing & mix!

Calories per bowl: 274 | Carbohydrate: 23g | Protein: 26 g | Fat: 8g

Middle Eastern Beef & Yogurt Pasta

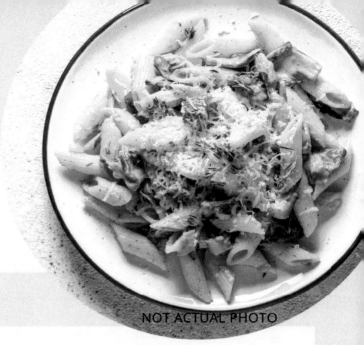

NOT ACTUAL PHOTO

SERVINGS: 5   PREPPING TIME: 15 MIN   COOKING TIME: 15 MIN

INGREDIENTS

- 250g Protein Pasta- I used <u>Kaizen.</u> You may use <u>Pastabilities</u>, or the Only Bean Black Bean Pasta.
- 1 cup fat free or low fat greek yogurt
- 1-2 tsp minced garlic
- 1/2 yellow onion, chopped
- 12 oz (3/4 lb) lean ground beef - I use 96/4
- 1 Tablespoon of 7 spice seasoning
- A bunch of chopped parsely
- Salt & Pepper to taste
- Option: Add chopped pine nuts

DIRECTIONS

1. Cook pasta according to box
2. In a spearate bowl, mix yogurt and minced garlic
3. On a pan cook chopped onion to brown
4. Add ground beef and 7 Spice seasoning and let simmer!
5. Drain pasta once cooked and toss into a large bowl
6. Add yogurt sauce and mix thoroughly
7. Add cooked beef and onion mixture and continue to toss
8. Finally, add chopped parsely!
9.

Calories per serving: 280 | Carbohydrate: 21g | Protein: 37g | Fat: 6g

Beef-less Stuffed Peppers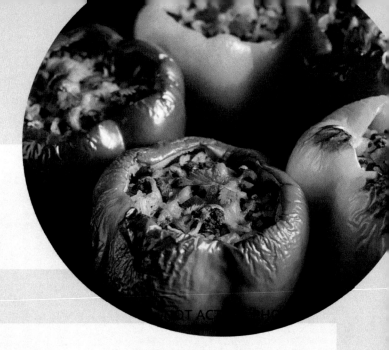

INGREDIENTS

- 3 large bell peppers (red, yellow, or orange)
- 1.5 package "Bee-less Grounds" "vegetarian beef" from Trader Joe's or (regular lean ground beef (1 lb)
- 1 1/4 cup Eggplant & Garlic Dip from Trader Joe's
- 1 package of shiratake rice (konjac) or Trader Joe's Riced Hearts of Palm.
- 1/4 cup Tomato paste
- 1/4 cup parsley, chopped
- Salt and Pepper to taste

DIRECTIONS

1. In a large bowl, combine Beefless Grounds, Eggplant dip, rice, tomato paste, parsley, salt & pepper. If using regular ground beef, cook beef on a pan first. Mix well and set aside.
2. Cut off the top of each bell pepper. Clear out the insides to make the pepper hollow
3. Spoon mixture into each pepper and place in a large pot.
4. Add water and tomato paste to the bottom of the pot.
5. Let simmer for 45 minutes until peppers are soft

Calories per serving: 180 | Carbohydrate: 30g | Protein: 20g | Fat: 6g

Spinach & Ricotta Stuffed Chicken

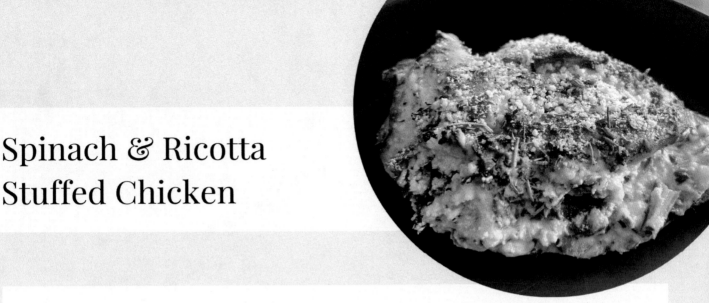

SERVINGS: 2-4   PREPPING TIME: 15 MIN   COOKING TIME: 15 MIN

INGREDIENTS

- 2 large chicken breasts (6-8 oz)
- 1/2 T olive oil to brush over chicken
- 1 tsp minced garlic
- 1/2 cup frozen spinach
- 1/2 cup part skim ricotta cheese
- 1/4 cup shredded lite mozzarella cheese
- 1/4 cup parmesan cheese
- 1/2 tsp paprika
- 1/2 tsp onion powder
- Salt & pepper to taste

Tip: I like the Salute Seasoning from Trader Joe's, but any of your favorite seasoning blend will work!

DIRECTIONS

1. Cook 1 tsp minced garlic on a pan over low heat. Make sure it doesn't burn.
2. Warm spinach in the microwave then pat dry
3. In a small bowl, mix ricotta, spinach, shredded mozzarella, salt and pepper
4. Brush chicken breasts with olive oil and season with salt, pepper, paprika, & onion powder.
5. Slice a pocket in each chicken breast
6. Spoon half the cheese mixture into each pocket. Pierce the pocket closed with a tooth pick
7. Place on parchment paper and airfry at 380F for 20 minutes or bake at 395F for 25 minutes.
8. With 5 minutes left, sprinkle the breasts with a T of parmesan cheese for a crispy crust

Calories per 6 oz chicken: 360 | Carbohydrate: 6g | Protein: 57g | Fat: 13g

Single Serving Low Carb Lasagna

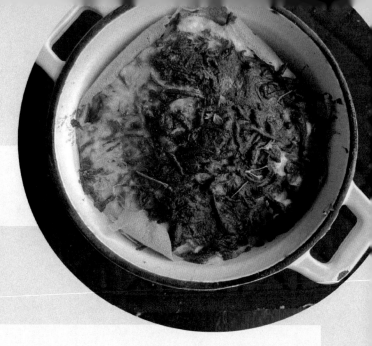

SERVINGS:1   PREPPING TIME: 10 MIN   COOKING TIME: 7 MIN

INGREDIENTS

- 1/4 cup part skim ricotta cheese
- 1/4 cup fat free cottage cheese
- 1 serving Calabrian Pasta Sauce (1/4 cup)
- 1.5 oz lite shredded mozzarella
- 1 egg wrap, sliced in quarters
- 1/4 cup Trader Joe's Meatless Grounds or 2 oz ground beef
- Italian seasoning

DIRECTIONS

1. Start by mixing the cottage cheese, the pasta sauce, Meatless Grounds and Italian seasoning in a bowl.
2. Cut one egg wrap into quarters.
3. Grease a small over safe bowl and place two of the egg wrap quarters at the bottom to cover the bottom.
4. Scoop 1/3 of the mixture on top.
5. Top it with a spoonfull of ricotta and a little mozzarella.
6. Repeat two more times!
7. Airfry at 350 for 7 minutes or until crispy or bake in the oven for 12 minutes at375F!

Calories per serving: 345 | Carbohydrate: 18g | **Protein:** 35g | Fat: 15g

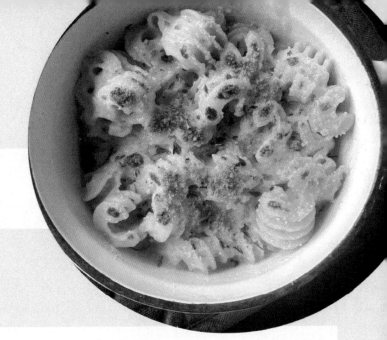

High-Protein Mac & Cheese ✅

SERVINGS: 2   PREPPING TIME: 2 MIN   COOKING TIME: 15-20 MIN

INGREDIENTS

- 1 serving Kaizen Noodles (250g)
- 1/2 up low fat or nonfat cottage cheese
- 1 oz fat-free cheddar cheese (or low fat)
- 1 baby bell of gouda (optional)
- 1/4 skim milk
- 1 T flour
- 20g Parmesan cheese
- 1-2 T powdered cheese
- Salt, pepper to taste
- Parsley flakes as garnish

DIRECTIONS

1. Make noodles per package instructions
2. Warm a separate pot over medium heat.
3. Blend cottage cheese before adding it to the pot. Once blended, add cottage cheese, cheddar, & parmesan and continue to stir.
4. Add the milk and continue to stir, allowing the liquid to evaporate, thickening the mixture.
5. Add flour and stir.
6. Once the cheese reaches a consistency you like, remove from heat.
7. Pour over noodles and stir.
8. Place mixture in an oversafe dish and broil for 3-5 minutes to crisp! Sprinkle with Parmensan and parsley flakes!

Calories per serving: 231 | Carbohydrate: 29g | **Protein: 18g** | Fat: 9g

Low-Carb Cauliflower "Mac" & Cheese 🌿

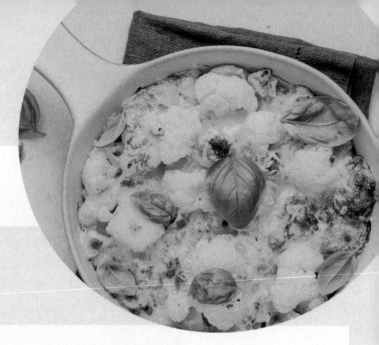

SERVINGS: 1   PREPPING TIME: 5 MIN   COOKING TIME: 15-20 MIN

INGREDIENTS

- 2 cups small cauliflower florets
- 1/2 cup low-fat cottage cheese (whipped/blended is best)
- 1/8 cup parmesan cheese
- 1/4 cup + 2 T light shredded 3 cheese blend (TJ's)
- 1 reduced fat sharp cheddar cheese slice, torn or 1 oz (1/4 cup) shredded
- 1 tsp mustard (Dijon works great)
- 1/2 tsp garlic powder
- 1/2 tsp onion powder
- Salt & pepper to taste
- Parsley for garnish

This can be used as a main dish, a side dish or a dip! Use riced cauliflower to create more of a dip-like consistency!

DIRECTIONS

1. In a baking dish or air fryer bin, toss 2 cups of small cauliflower florets. Spray with avocado oil then season with salt and pepper.
2. Airfry for 10 minutes at 350F or bake for 15 min at 375F
3. In a medium sized bowl, mix the cottage cheese (blend with an immersion blender or in a blender for smoother consistency), parmesan, shredded cheese, mustard, onion, garlic, salt & pepper then mix
4. Once cauliflower is baked, mix in with cheese and pour into an oven safe dish (5-6inch).
5. Sprinkle with 2 T shredded cheese and smoked paprika then cover with foil.
6. Airfry for 15 min at 350F or bake for 30 at 375. When there is 5 minutes left, remove the foil from dish to create a crusted top.

Calories: 340 | Carbohydrate: 15g | **Protein: 38g** | Fat: 14g

Low-Carb Cottage Cheese Alfredo Pasta

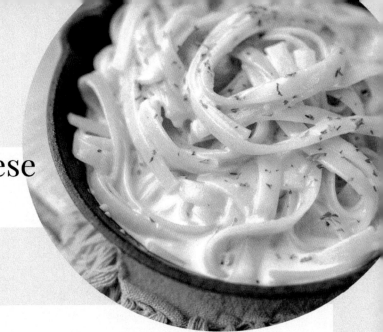

SERVINGS: 2   PREPPING TIME: 10 MIN   COOKING TIME: 15 MIN

INGREDIENTS

- 1 package Hearts of Palm Noodles (Palmini or Trader Joe's)
- 1 cup fat free milk
- 3/4 cup fat free cottage cheese (you can use low fat too)
- 1 T cornstarch (optional- if omitted reduce milk to 1/2 cup)
- 1/2 tsp garlic powder
- 1/4 cup + 2 T parmesan cheese
- 1/4 tsp dried basil & dried oregano
- 1/4 tsp onion salt (or onion powder)
- Salt & Pepper to taste
- handful of chopped parsley

I love to add broccoli, spinach or peas to this dish!

DIRECTIONS

1. Blend all ingredients, except for pasta and basil and oregano in a blender or food processor. I just use a cup blender :)
2. Pour mixture into a saucepan over medium heat.
3. Add pasta, basil, and oregano & cover
4. Let cook form 5-7 minutes, stirring occasionally as the liquid gets thicker.

Calories per serving 403 | Carbohydrate: 24g | **Protein: 47g** | Fat: 13g

My Favorite Healthy Meatloaf

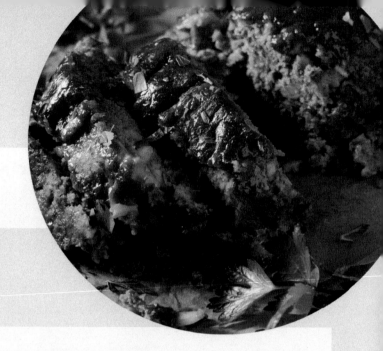

SERVINGS: 4   PREPPING TIME: 15 MIN   COOKING TIME: 60 MIN

INGREDIENTS

- 1/4 cup plus 2 tbsp ketchup, I use organic - you can also mix in BBQ
- 2 tsp Worcestershire sauce
- 1/2 small onion, minced (1 cup)
- 2-3 stalks of Carrot, chopped
- 3 leaves of kale, chopped
- 1/2 cup peas
- 1.3 lb 99% lean ground turkey
- 1 tsp olive oil
- 1/2 cup seasoned whole wheat or gluten-free breadcrumbs (or Quest Chips/ Snack House Puffs)
- 1 large egg
- 1 tsp salt
- 1-2 tsp Garlic Powder
- Parsley for garnish

DIRECTIONS

1. Preheat the oven to 350F.
2. In a small bowl combine 2 tbsp of the ketchup with Worcestershire sauce.
3. In a small skillet, heat olive oil and saute chopped carrots and onion on low heat until onions are translucent for 3 to 5 minutes, then remove from heat.
4. In a medium bowl combine the turkey, onion, carrots, peas, kale, breadcrumbs, egg, 1/4 cup ketchup, garlic powder, and salt.
5. Place mixture into a loaf pan or shape into a loaf and place on a baking pan. Spoon 2 T ketchup sauce on top!
6. Bake uncovered for 55-60 minutes, then let sit to cool. Top with chopped parsley!

Calories per serving: 292 | Carbohydrate: 32g | **Protein:** 35g | Fat: 1g

My Favorite Low Carb Bean-less Chili

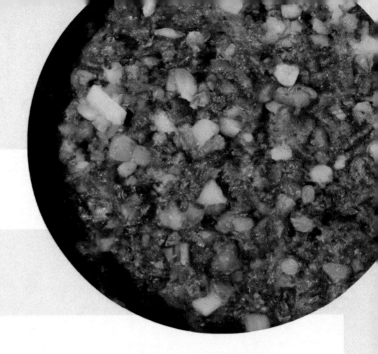

SERVINGS: 6   PREPPING TIME: 15 MIN   COOKING TIME: 60 MIN

INGREDIENTS

- 1 lb Lean ground beef / lean ground turkey / lean ground chicken or "Beef-less" Vegan Beef
- 1 yellow or red onion
- 1-2 cloves garlic
- 1/2 T butter
- 3 bell peppers or 1 bag of small sweet mini peppers
- 1 large can fire roasted diced tomatoes
- 4-5 Carrots or half bag of baby carrots
- 1-2 cups bone broth or beef/chicken broth/ vegetable broth
- a bunch of kale or other leafy green
- 1 scoop of Greek yogurt for garnish
- 1-2 bag of Sloppy Joe Mix

Sloppy Joe Mix Alternative:
- 1 ½1/2 teaspoons kosher salt
- 1/2 teaspoon ground black pepper
- 1 tablespoon oregano
- 1 tablespoon ground chili powder
- 2 teaspoons ground cumin
- 1 1/2 teaspoons ground chipotle chili powder
- 1 1/2 teaspoons garlic powder
- 1/2 teaspoon ground cinnamon

DIRECTIONS

1. Melt butter at the bottom of a large pot
2. Add onions, garlic, and meat and cook on medium until meat is browned and onions are translucent.
3. Add spices or 1-2 bags of Sloppy Joe seasoning mixture and stir. Taste to ensure flavor is to your liking. Some prefer 2 bags over 1.
4. Add broth, vegetables (except kale), and canned tomatoes & continuously stir. Bring chili to a boil and then reduce heat and let simmer.
5. If you want a thicker chili, let it simmer with the lid partially open for another 20-30 minutes so liquid evaporates.
6. About five minutes before it's finished cooking, add in any leafy greens
7. Serve and top with cheese or Greek yogurt!

Calories per serving with 96% beef, no garnish : 206 | Carbohydrate: 22g | Protein: 23g | Fat: 3g

Low-Calorie Spring Rolls with High-Protein Peanut Sauce ✅

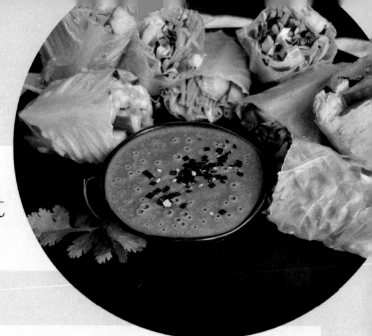

SERVINGS: 8 TOTAL HALVES   PREPPING TIME: 15 MIN   COOKING TIME: 5 MIN IF COOKING SHRIMP

INGREDIENTS

- 26 cooked shrimp (100g) or tofu
- 4 rice paper sheets
- 2 Persian cucumbers, julienned
- 1/2 cup shredded carrots
- 1/2 cup shredded cabbage
- Romaine lettuce leaves

Sauce:

- 6 T Pb2 Powder (3 servings)
- 2 T Soy Sauce
- 1 T honey
- Grated Ginger (optional)

DIRECTIONS

1. If shrimp isn't pre-cooked, cook shrimp with your preferred method.
2. Prepare spring roll ingredients
3. Wet each rice paper roll and place it on a flat, clean surface.
4. Place romaine leaf face up directly in the middle of the wrap.
5. Fill with cabbage, carrots, cucumbers, and shrimp. Optional to add avocado!
6. Top with another romaine leaf to hold all in place then slice each roll in half.
7. Begin by rolling the rice paper like a burrito - fold in the ends.
8. In a small bowl, mix PB2, soy sauce, honey, and grated ginger. Mix with water!
9. Dip each half in dressing and enjoy!

Calories per half with sauce: 60 | Carbohydrate: 9g | **Protein: 5g** | Fat: 1g

Calories for entire sauce: 260 | Carbohydrate: 35g | **Protein: 20g** | Fat: 5g

Sushi Cups

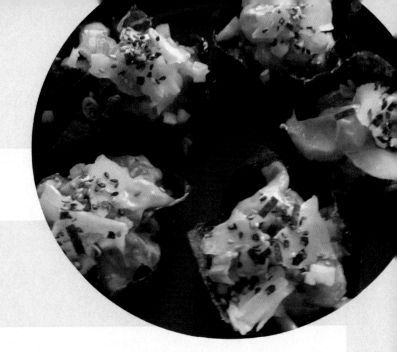

SERVINGS: 12 CUPS   PREPPING TIME: 15 MIN   <u>COOKING TIME: 30 MIN</u>

INGREDIENTS

- 6 oz fresh salmon, chopped
- 3 Nori Seaweed Sheets
- 1 cup white rice, cooked
- 1 T Soy Sauce or Coconut Aminos
- 1 tsp Sesame Oil
- Furikake Seasoning
- 1 chopped Persian Cucumber
- 1 sprig chopped green onion
- 3 T sushi ginger (or more!)

Sauce:

- 3-4 T Lite Mayonaise
- 1-2 T Sriracha to taste

DIRECTIONS

1. Boil white rice according to package.
2. Chop fresh salmon into cubes and place them in a bowl.
3. Add 1 tsp sesame oil, soy sauce, and furikake seasoning to bowl and stir. Set aside.
4. In a separate bowl mix mayonaise and siracha to make a spicy mayo.
5. Chop cucumbers and green onion and set aside.
6. Take Nori sheets and tear along the dotted line to create quarters.
7. Spray a muffin tin with oil.
8. Place a tablespoon or 15g of white rice on a quarter of a nori sheet and place inside a muffin slot. Add salmon and repeat for 12 muffin slots.
9. Place muffin tin in the oven for 20 minutes at 400F until Nori is crispy.
10. Once cups are cooked, dress with ginger, cucumber, onion, mayo and more furikake seasoning!

Calories for each 115 | Carbohydrate: 8g | Protein: 7g | Fat: 6g

Easy Sushi Wrap

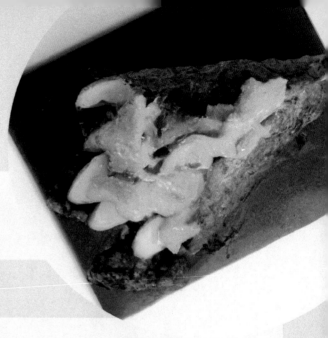

SERVINGS: 1 WRAP   PREPPING TIME: 10 MIN   COOKING TIME: 0 MIN UNLESS
COOKING SHRIMP - 7

INGREDIENTS

- 1 Nori Seaweed Sheet
- 5 large cooked shrimp
- 1/2 Persian cucumber, sliced thin
- 1 T Sushi Ginger

Sauce:

- 1 tsp siracha sauce
- 1 T light Mayonaise
- 1 T Soy Sauce
- Furikake Seasoning

DIRECTIONS

1. Cook shrimp if they are not cooked already.
2. Make the spicy mayo sauce by mixing sriracha, mayo, furikake seasoning and soy sauce.
3. Lay a nori sheet on a flat surface and slice a slit from the center of the sheet to the edge of the sheet (like a clock hand).
4. Smear the spicy mayo on the bottom left portion of the nori sheet, to the left of the slit.
5. Chop cooked shrimp and place it directly above the sauce, in the top left quadrant.
6. Chop cucumbers and lay them out gently in the top right quadrant of the nori sheet.
7. Add ginger to the bottom right quadrant, the last quadrant and to the right of the slit.
8. Fold from the bottom left quadrant up, then right, then down to form a layered triangle. Enjoy!

Calories: 150 | Carbohydrate: 7g | Protein: 20g | Fat: 5g

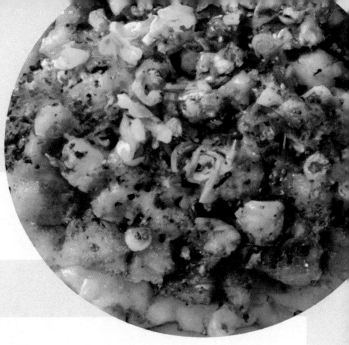

High-Protein Waffle Crispy Rice

SERVINGS: 2   PREPPING TIME: 10 MIN   COOKING TIME: 17-20 MIN

INGREDIENTS

- 1.5 cups cauliflower rice, dried!
- 1/4 cup cooked & drained Kaizen Protein Rice (You can also use Banza, but it will contain less protein.
- 1/2 Persian cucumber, sliced thin
- 2 T egg whites
- 2 T all-purpose flour
- 2 T Furikake seasoning
- 1 tsp Sesame Oil
- 1 T Sushi Ginger
- 2 sheets of toasted seaweed snack
- 1 stem of green onion, chopped
- 4 oz Sashimi Grade Salmon, Tuna or Simply Surimi Crab Stick

Sauce:
- 2 tsp siracha sauce
- 2 T light mayonnaise
- 2-3 T truffle Soy Sauce
- Furikake Seasoning

DIRECTIONS

1. Ensure your cauliflower rice is dry. Pat it dry or cook out the water as best as you can.
2. Cook and drain the protein rice.
3. Combine both rice with egg whites, flour, 1 T furikake seasoning
4. Grease your waffle maker with 1 tsp of sesame oil, or any oil.
5. Spread rice mixture out onto hot waffle maker and shut closed. Let cook for 5 minutes.
6. While the rice is cooking, mix your fish with lite mayonaise, sriracha, soy sauce, chopped cucumber, torn seaweed, sushi ginger green onion.
7. Once rice looks cooked and slightly golden, remove the rice from waffle maker and place in the airfryer for 6-7 minutes at 380F or bake in the oven for 10 minutes at 350F.
8. Spread fish mixture on top of the crispy rice waffle and enjoy!

Calories per serving with salmon: 296 | Carbohydrate: 20g | Protein: 28g | Fat: 11g

Lavash Bread Pizza

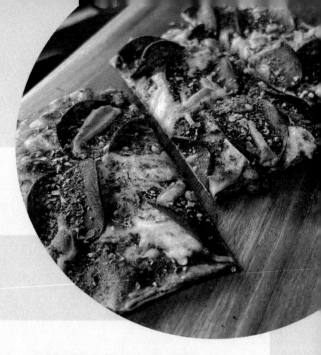

SERVINGS: 2   PREPPING TIME: 10 MIN   COOKING TIME: 8 MIN

INGREDIENTS

- 2 sheets of Lavash Bread
- 2 wedges laughing cow cheese
- 2-3 T pizza sauce
- 1.5oz or 1/2 c shredded light mozzarella cheese
- Pizza seasoning or Italian seasoning
- Cheesy seasoning
- Oregano
- Applegate Turkey Pepperoni

DIRECTIONS

1. Preheat oven to 350 degrees Fahrenheit.
2. Spray parchment paper with avocado oil & place on an oven tray.
3. Place 2 sheets of lavash bread on paper on the tray. Spray with avocado oil.
4. Heat for 3-4 minutes.
5. Take out, spread laughing cow cheese on both sheets.
6. Smear 1-2 T of pizza sauce.
7. Sprinkle MOST of the cheese on each sheet.
8. Add all seasoning & turkey pepperoni then broil for another 3-4 minutes.

Calorie for ONE Pizza: 250 Carbohydrate: 17, Protein: 23, Fat: 10
Recipe Makes 2

White Sauce Lavash Pizza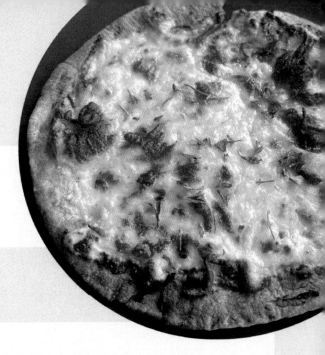

SERVINGS: 1   PREPPING TIME: 10 MIN   COOKING TIME: 12 MIN

INGREDIENTS

- 1 lavash pita (I used Josephs but you can also use a high-protein tortilla)
- 1/4 cup low-fat cottage cheese, blended (50g)
- 1/2 tsp minced garlic
- 1 lite laughing cow cheese wedge
- 1 heaping T parmesan cheese
- 1/4 cup reduced fat mozzarella
- Herbs de Provence or italian seasoning
- Nutritional Yeast or Cheesy sprinkle (TJ)
- Salt & pepper to taste
- 1 tsp olive oil
- Dried parsley for garnish

DIRECTIONS

1. Preheat bread for 2 minutes in airfryer or oven at 375F.
2. Mix cottage cheese, garlic, laughing cow cheese wedge, parmesan cheese, nutritional yeast, Herbs de Provence, salt & pepper.
3. Pour mixture overbread and spread out, leaving 1/2 inch of space around the edges.
4. Drizzle 1 tsp olive oil on top.
5. Place in the airfryer at 380 for 10 minutes of the oven at 400 for 12 minutes or until golden and crisp.
6. Sprinkle with dried parsley!

Calorie for ONE Pizza: 222 Carbohydrate: 14 | Protein: 21 | Fat: 9

Crispy Salmon & Cheese Taco

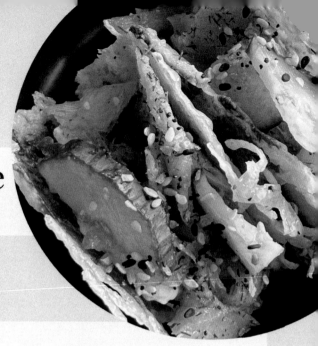

SERVINGS: 4 TACOS   PREPPING TIME: 7 MIN   COOKING TIME: 5 MIN

INGREDIENTS

- 2 oz (1/2 cup) lite shredded mozzarella
- 2 oz (1/2 cup) shredded parmesan
- 2 slices smoked Dillicious Salmon or Everything but the Bagel Seasoned Salmon
- 8 T low fat cottage cheese (2T each taco)
- A handful of sliced cucumbers, small
- Everything but the Bagel Seasoning

DIRECTIONS

1. Grease a pan with some avocado oil and turn on medium heat.
2. Mix shredded mozzarella and shredded parmesan in a bowl then sprinkle 1 oz of mixture onto pan and spread into a disc shape. Repeat 3 more times
3. Cover pan and let cheese melt and brown. You may sprinkle with EBTB seasoning.
4. Once golden, use a spatula to remove from pan and place over small cucumber or bottle to dry and harden into a taco shape
5. Once hard, add cottage cheese, salmon, cucumbers, and seasoning!

Calorie per taco: 160 | Carbohydrate: 4g | Protein: 21g | Fat: 6g

Trader Joe's Mediterranean Bowl ✔

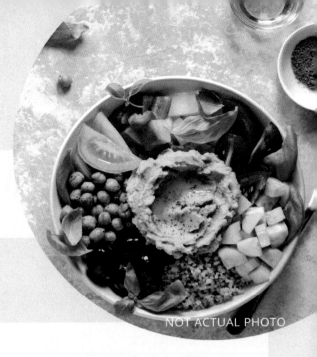

NOT ACTUAL PHOTO

SERVINGS: 1   **PREPPING TIME: 5 MIN**   **COOKING TIME: 10 MIN**

INGREDIENTS

- 1 serving (4 oz) Chicken Shawarma Chicken Thighs or frozen Beef Kebobs or Hi-Protein Veggie Burger (All from Trader Joe's!)
- 1 package of hearts of palm rice
- A handful of spring mix
- 1/ 4 cup Middle Eastern Chickpea Salad
- 1/2 oz sliced kalamata olives
- 2 T hummus
- 1.5 oz (1/4 cup) fat-free feta
- 2 T Creamy Garlic & Cucumber Tzatiki Dip
- 2 T Green Goddess Dressing

DIRECTIONS

1. Choose which protein you'd like to use and cook according to package
2. Warm the hearts of palm rice on a skillet or in the microwave & place into a large bowl or dinner plate
3. Add chickpea salad, olives, hummus, feta, Tzatziki Dip and protein.
4. Drizzle with Green Goddess dressing!

Ways to Alter this meal:
1. Chicken breast to bring calories down
2. Mix or replace hearts of palm with regular rice or cauliflower rice if you don't like hearts of palm rice

Calories: 488 | Carbohydrate: 33 | Protein: 38 | Fat: 23

Taco Casserole ✅

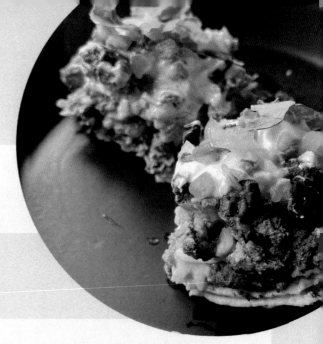

SERVINGS: 6 SQUARES   PREPPING TIME: 10 MIN   COOKING TIME: 12 MIN

INGREDIENTS

- 3 sheet sof Lavash bread
- 12 oz 96% lean beef or plant beef
- 1/4 cup chopped onion
- 1 packet of taco seasoning
- 3 oz fat free cheese
- 3 laughing cow

Topping Ideas:

- 2 oz black olives
- 1/2 cup fat free Greek yogurt
- 1/2 cup pico de gallo
- Chopped lettuce
- Taco sauce

DIRECTIONS

1. Start by greasing a pan and cooking 3/4 of a lb (12 oz) of lean ground beef with a quarter cup of onion and one packet of taco seasoning.
2. While the beef is cooking, spread, one wedge of Lite Laughing Cow Cheese on one side of a Lavash sheet.
3. Place 3 1/2 to 4 ounces of ground beef mixture onto lavash sheet then add 1 oz of fat free shredded cheese
4. Repeat step 3 two more times to create three layers.
5. Bake in the oven for 10 to 12 minutes at 400°F
6. Once finished, add your favorite toppings like fresh salsa, more cheese, sliced black olives, taco sauce, and low fat sour cream, or fat-free Greek yogurt.
7. Slice into six squares and enjoy.

Calorie per square: 150 | Carbohydrate: 10g | Protein: 19g | Fat:4g

Sweet Pepper Nachos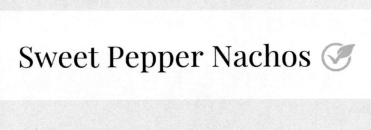

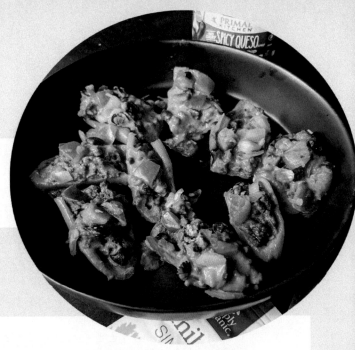

SERVINGS: 1-2   PREPPING TIME: 12 MIN   COOKING TIME: 15-20 MIN

INGREDIENTS

- 1/2 bag of sweet peppers, halve
- ground lean meat (chicken, turkey, or 96/4 lean beef (Trader Joe's or Laura's!) or Plant Beef
- Primal Kitchen SPicy Nacho dip
- Simply Organic Simmer Sauce (or fave taco seasoning)
- 1/2 cup black beans

DIRECTIONS

1. Slice sweet pepper in half and lay on a sheet of foil.
2. Cook meat with simmer sauce or seasoning until cooked through.
3. Once meat is cooked, spoon into sweet peppers, trying to fit each spoonfull into each pepper (but also not totally necessary).
4. Top with some black beans!
5. Airfry for 15 min at 400F or bake at 425 for 18 minutes
6. Once cooked and crispy, top with fresh toppings like: tomatoes or pico de gallo, guacamole, lettuce.

Calories: Variable

Cilantro Lime Shrimp Tacos

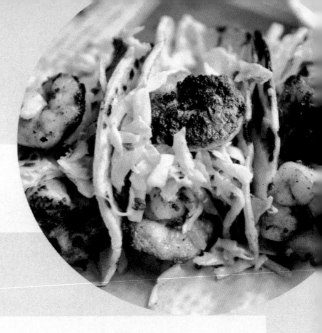

SERVINGS: 1
(3 SMALL TACOS)

PREPPING TIME: 10 MIN

COOKING TIME: 5 MIN

INGREDIENTS

- 9 large shrimp
- Small Tortillas: TJ's Jicama Wraps or Carb Savvy Tortillas / Mission Tortillas
- 1 Cup shredded cabbage slaw
- 1/2 cup Trader Joe's Cilantro Salad Dressing or Primal Kitchen Cilantro Lime Dressing OR Bolthouse Farms Cilantro Avocado Dressing
- 1/2 lime

Slaw Sauce:

- 3 T Taco Sauce
- 1 T 0% Fat Greek Yogurt

DIRECTIONS

1. If cooking shrimp, cook on a pan with paprika and a spray of avocado oil. You may also microwave for faster cook time.

2. Place shredded cabbage in a bowl. Mix 3 T taco sauce with 1 T greek yogurt. Stir until cabbage is coated.

3. Lay 3 tortillas out flat and place mixed cabbage in the center of each.

4. Place 3 large shrimp on each taco & drizzle cilantro dressing on top

5. Squeeze lime on tacos and enjoy!

Per Taco:

Calories: 85 | Carbohydrate: 5 grams, Protein: 10 grams, Fat: 3 grams

Total for 3:

Calories: 255 | Carbohydrate: 15 grams, Protein: 30 grams, Fat: 9 grams

---

Beef Tostada

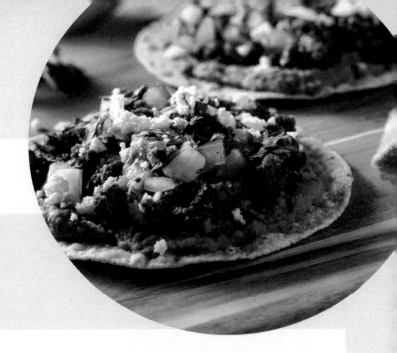

INGREDIENTS

- 1 lb 96% lean ground beef, but you'll use 2 oz
- 1/2 cup enchilada sauce (for 1lb beef)
- 1 packet of taco seasoning (for 1lb beef)
- 1 carb savy tortilla
- 1/4 cup fat free refried beans
- 1/4 + 1/8 cup light Mexican blend cheese
- 1 T mild pico de Gallo
- 1 green onion chopped
- 1/4 cup fat free greek yogurt as a topping
- 1/2 oz sliced black olives

DIRECTIONS

1. Cook a lb of lean beef with enchilada sauce and taco seasoning!
2. Airfry or bake the tortilla for 3-4 min at 380F to harden it.
3. Mix 2 oz beef, cheese, and beans. Once tortilla is warm, smear mixture on top.
4. Airfry again for 4 minutes.
5. Top with 1/8 cup shredded cheese
6. Airfry for another 1 minute to melt cheese
7. Tortilla should be crispy! Once cooked, top with pico de gallo, olives, onions, and a Greek yogurt dollop!
8. Optional to add avocado (more calories!)
9. Enjoy!

Calories: 280 | Carbohydrate: 20g | Protein: 28 g | Fat: 10 g

Taco Bowl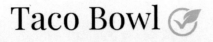

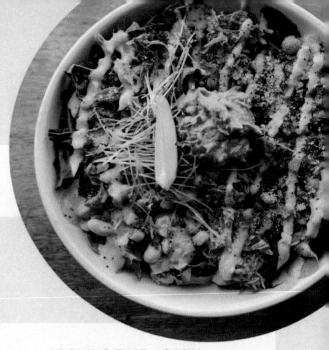

SERVINGS: 1	PREPPING TIME: 5 MIN	COOKING TIME: 10 MIN

INGREDIENTS

- 1 cup Spicy Mexican Cauliflower Rice or regular cauliflower rice
- 1/2 cup roasted corn
- 1/2 cup fire bell peppers
- 1/2 onion
- Romaine hearts- chopped
- 3.5 oz 96% lean beef or plant beef
- 1 packet of taco seasoning
- 1/4 c nonfat Greek yogurt
- 1 oz lite shredded Mexican cheese
- 1 cup fresh salsa or chopped tomato
- Taco sauce
- Lime wedge
- Salt & pepper to taste
- Optional: Fat-free refried beans, avocado/guac (will increase calorie count)

DIRECTIONS

Spray a pan with oil and warm to medium heat. Cook cauliflower rice, corn and peppers in the pan, if frozen.

2. In a separate pan, combine chopped onion, beef, and taco seasoning & cook, mixing throughout the cooking process.

3. Chop romaine lettuce and place in a bowl.

4. Once cooked, layer cauliflower mixture & beef in a bowl over chopped romaine.

5. Add cheese, salsa, greek yogurt and any other toppings you wish to include.

6. Drizzle with taco sauce & lime.

Calories: 397 | Carbohydrate: 31g | Protein: 45g | Fat: 11g

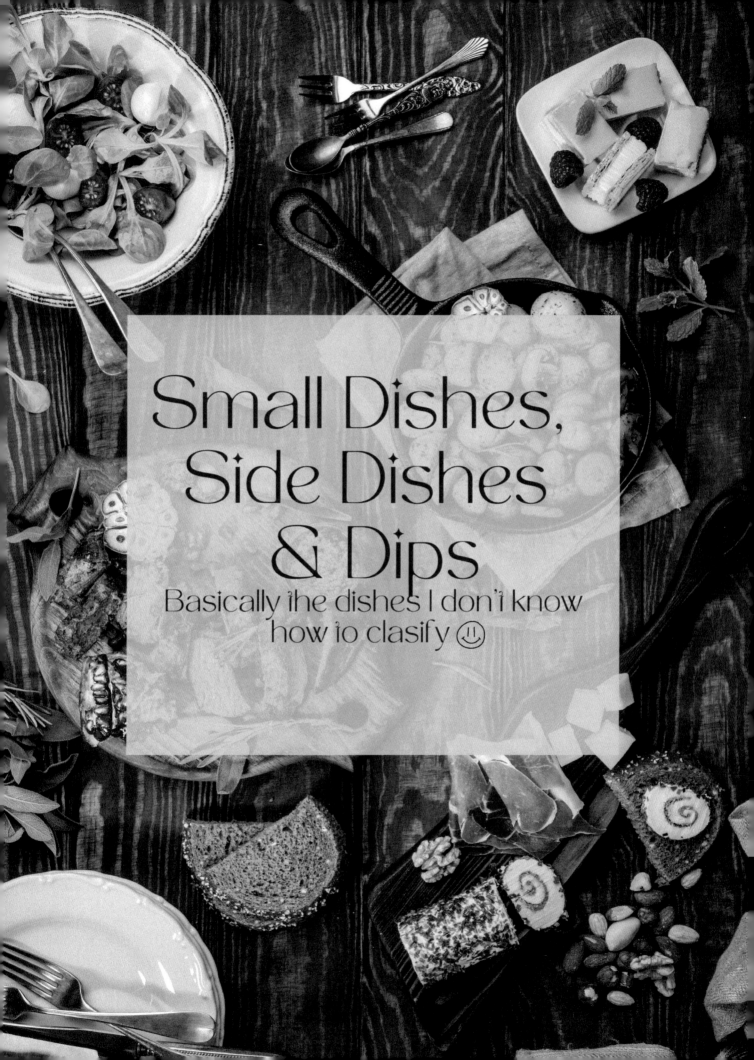

Small Dishes, Side Dishes & Dips

Basically the dishes I don't know
how to clasify 😊

Mediterranean Side Salad ✅

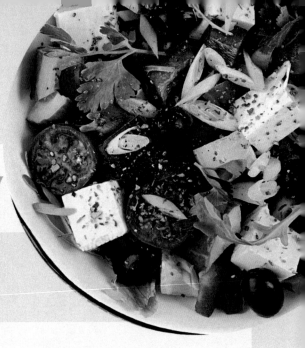

| SERVINGS: 1 | PREPPING TIME: 5 MIN | COOKING TIME: 0 MIN |

INGREDIENTS

- 1 cup (22g) mixed greens
- 2 oz (56g) fat-free feta cheese
- 1/8 small red onion, sliced
- 2 tbsp (20g) green olives
- 1/2 medium vine ripe tomato, sliced
- 1 small cucumber, sliced
- 1 T olive oil - OR swap for 2 T low fat Italian if desired
- Handful chopped parsley
- Salt and pepper to taste

Optional: toasted pita chips

DIRECTIONS

1. Combine mixed greens, feta cheese, red onion, green olives, tomatoes, cucumbers.
2. Drizzle with olive oil and add salt and pepper to taste.

With Olive Oil: 280 calories , Carbohydrate: 13 g, Protein: 16 g, Fat: 20 g
With Low Fat Italian: 197 calories, Carbohydrate: 16 g, Protein: 16 g, Fat: 8 g

High-Protein Hashbrown Fritters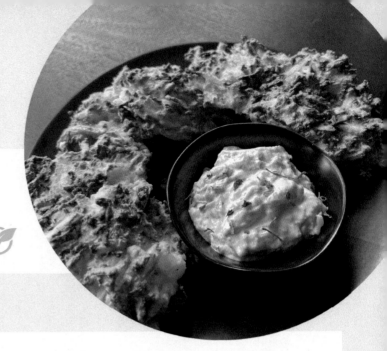

SERVINGS: 7 FRITTERS   **PREPPING TIME: 10 MIN**   **COOKING TIME: 10 MIN**

INGREDIENTS

- 6 oz Trader Joe's Frozen Hashbrowns
- 1.5 oz lite Mexican blend cheese (1/4 cup + 1/8 cup)
- 1/2 scoop <u>Quest All Purpose protein powder</u>
- 3 T liquid egg whites
- Trader Joe's Caramelized Onion Dip (Vegan or Regular!)

DIRECTIONS

1. Mix hashbrowns, cheese, protein powder together then add egg whites until it creates a thick consistency
2. Form into small discs and place in an airfryer (or oven) for 10 min at 380F in the airfryer or oven with 2 min broil at the end.
3. Plate and dip with Trader Joe's Carmelized Onion dip!

To make your own Caramelized Onion Dip:

- Cook 1 cup of onions on a skillet over medium heat until golden brown and jam like. Add a T of water every so often to keep from burning.
- Whisk 1/4 cup lowfat greek yogurt, 1/2 cup low fat sour cream, and 1/4 cup low fat cream cheese. Mix in 1/2 tsp garlic and onion powder, 1/4 tsp balsamic vinegar, and a pinch of salt.
- Add the onions, stir, and refrigerate!

Calories for 7 patties: 300 | Carbohydrate: 28g | Protein: 33g | Fat: 6g

Protein Naan Bread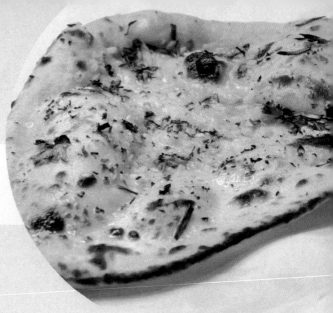

SERVINGS: 2   PREPPING TIME: 10 MIN   COOKING TIME: 10 MIN

INGREDIENTS

- 100 g All-Purpose Flour or Gluten Free Flour
- 50g casein protein powder or multipurpose protein powder
- 125g 0% Greek yogurt
- 5g baking powder
- Garlic powder
- Salt to taste
- 5g nutritional yeast for cheese flavor
- 1 tsp butter to spread
- Dried parsley for topping

DIRECTIONS

1. Mix flour, protein, baking powder, garlic, and salt (dry ingredients) in a bowl.
2. Add Greek yogurt and mix well using your hands to create a dough ball.
3. Flour a cutting board or counter top, and divide the dough into 4 pieces, roilled out.
4. Heat a skillet with 1/2 tsp butter and cook each piece evenly on both sides
5. Melt half a tsp of butter and brush on each.
6. Sprinkle nutritional yeast and salt on top and enjoy!

Calories per serving: 218 | Carbohydrate: 24g | Protein: 17g | Fat: 6g

Protein Garlic Cheesey Bread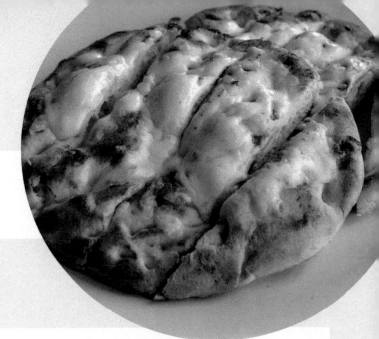

SERVINGS: 1-2   PREPPING TIME: 5 MIN   COOKING TIME:7 MIN

INGREDIENTS

- 2 high protein tortillas (<u>Hero</u> is great here because it's fluffier)
- 1 slice of light cheddar
- 1 wedgeof lite Laughing cow cheese square
- 1/4 low fat mozzarella
- 1 tsp minced garlic
- 1/2 tsp onion salt
- optional: jalapeño, chopped olives

DIRECTIONS

1. Lay out both tortillas on a flat working surface.
2. Smear the laughing cow cheese wedge on both.
3. Cut up the lite cheese slice into 4 pieces and place over one totrilla.
4. On the other tortilla, spread the low fat mozzarella cheese
5. Sprinkle minced garlic over the mozzarella cheese shreds and top with onion salt and cheesey seasoning.
6. Place the seasoned totrilla with the shredded mozzarella on top of the other tortilla.
7. Air fry for 7 minutes at 380°F

Calories for entire bread: 411 | Carbohydrate: 36g | Protein: 34 g | Fat: 15 g

High Protein, Low Carb Jicama Fries ✅

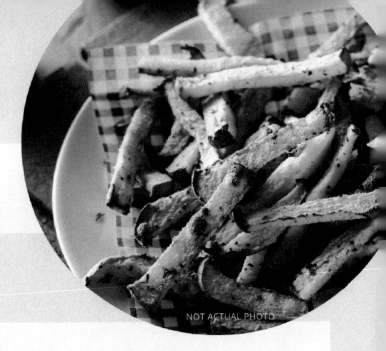

NOT ACTUAL PHOTO

SERVINGS: 1   PREPPING TIME: 5 MIN   COOKING TIME: 8 MIN

INGREDIENTS

- 3 servings of jicama spears, pre-sliced from Trader Joes'!
- 1 package of SnackHouse Keto Puffs - fiery hot flavor (Code: PROTEINSNACKQUEEN
- 1 spray of avocado oil
- Ketchup or favorite dipping sauce

Get 15% off SnackHouse Puffs with code #PROETINSNACKQUEEN

DIRECTIONS

1. Make a small slit in the protein puff bag to let air out.
2. Crush the puffs with a rolling pin or water bottle.
3. Sprinkle crushed puffs over jicama slices and toss with hands.
4. Spray one spray of avocado oil and continue to toss until all spears are coated
5. Air fry at 380°F for 8 min!
6. Dip in ketchup & ENJOY!

Calories: 212 | Carbohydrate: 23g | Protein: 19g | Fat: 5g

Crispy Carrots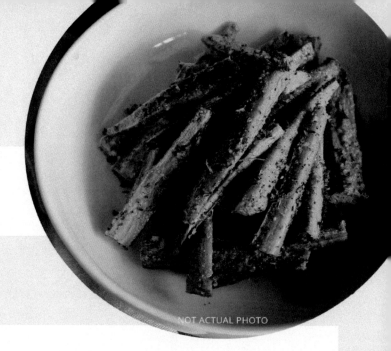

NOT ACTUAL PHOTO

SERVINGS: 3   **PREPPING TIME: 10 MIN**   **COOKING TIME: 30 MIN**

INGREDIENTS

- 1 lb carrots, peeled & julienned or sliced thin
- 2 T olive oil
- 2/3 cup parmesan cheese
- 1 T cornstarch
- 1.5 tsp onion powder
- 1.5 tsp garlic powder
- salt & papper to taste
- chopped parsley for garnish

Recommended Sauces:

ranch, ketchup, spicy mayo

DIRECTIONS

1. Preheat the oven to 400°F
2. In a bowl, mix oil, 1/3 cup parmesan, cornstarch, onion powder, garlic powder, salt, and pepper. Mix well.
3. Toss in carrots and continue to mix until carrots are coated.
4. Spread carrots evenly in a single layer on a baking sheet.
5. Bake in oven for 25 minutes, flipping carrots half way.
6. At 25 minutes, sprinkle the last 1/3 cup of parmesan on top to create a thin layer of melted, crispy cheese.
7. Bake for another 5 minutes.
8. Garnish with parsely and enjoy!

Calories per serving: 242 | Carbohydrate: 17g | Protein: 7g | Fat: 15g

Buffalo Chicken Dip

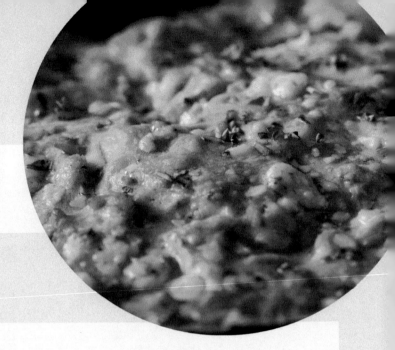

SERVINGS: 2   PREPPING TIME: 10 MIN   COOKING TIME: 25

INGREDIENTS

- 6 oz shredded chicken breast - (use rotisserie chicken for faster prep!)
- 1 1/2 cup 0% *fat free* greek yogurt
- 1.5 oz lite cream cheese
- 2 oz low fat shredded cheese
- 4 T buffalo sauce or to taste- I used New Primal
- 1 T ranch seasoning
- Topping: 1 oz/ 1/4 cup low fat shredded cheese
- Chopped green onion

DIRECTIONS

1. Mix yogurt & cream cheese along with ranch seasoning and buffalo sauce
2. Toss in a blender or immersion blend mixture.
3. Preheat oven to 350°F
4. Prep shredded chicken in a baking dish.
5. Pour mixture over chicken.
6. Top with 1 oz of shredded cheese.
7. Place baking dish in the oven for 20 minutes. Broil for 3-5 minutes.
8. Chop a handful of green onion and set aside.
9. Once done, sprinkle onions, let cool then enjoy!

Calories per serving: 314 | Carbohydrate: 13g | Protein: 43 g | Fat: 11g

Spinach Artichoke & Chicken Dip

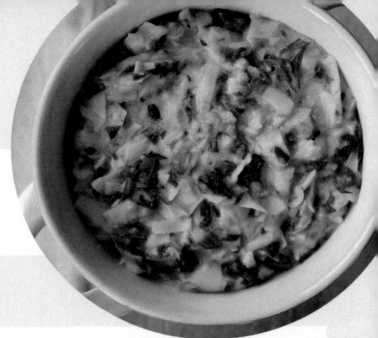

SERVINGS: 1-2   **PREPPING TIME: 10 MIN**   **COOKING TIME: 30-35**

INGREDIENTS

- 8 oz artichoke hearts (usually use just under 1 can)
- 1/4 cup parmesan cheese
- 1/4 cup shredded lite mozzarella cheese + 2 T
- 4 oz pre-cooked chicken breast filets, chopped or shredded
- 1/4 cup fat-free cottage cheese
- 1/2 cup fat free Greek yogurt
- 1/2 tsp garlic powder
- 1/2 cup spinach, frozen or fresh
- Salt & pepper to taste
- Sprinke of low fat shredded mozzarella cheese
- Parsley for garnish

DIRECTIONS

1. If baking, preheat your oven to 375F
2. Grease a small-medium-sized baking dish.
3. Blend parmesan cheese, cottage cheese, garlic, and greek yogurt in a blender or in a bowl using an immersion blender
4. Drain the artichoke hearts well and mix them in the cheese mixture with dry chopped spinach. Add chicken & continue to mix.
5. Pour mixture into baking dish. Sprinkle with low fat mozzarella cheese.
6. Bake for 15 minutes at 375 of airfry at 350°F for 9-10 min

Make this vegetarian by omitting the chicken! It will still be high protein!

Calories per serving: 418 | Carbohydrate: 13g | Protein: 60 g | Fat: 14g

Elote Dip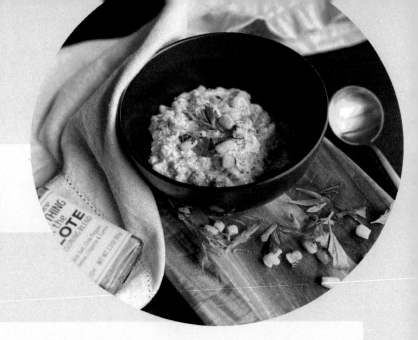

SERVINGS:1-2   PREPPING TIME: 5 MIN   COOKING TIME:
                                                    5 IF COOKING CORN

INGREDIENTS

- 1 cup roasted corn - I used the frozen Fire Roasted Corn from Trader Joe's! You can use canned.
- 1/3 cup fat free greek yogurt
- 1/2 cup fat free or low-fat cottage cheese
- A lot of Everything But the Elote Seasoning (2-3 T)
- 1/4 cup 1 T or 1.5 oz fat-free Feta cheese
- A handful of chopped cilantro

DIRECTIONS

1. Heat the corn on a skillet or in a microwave to save time!
2. Add yogurt, cottage cheese and seasoning to a bowl or blender. Immersion blend or blend in a small blender.
3. Add feta, corn, chopped cilantro, and mix!

Calories per serving: 300 | Carbohydrate: 34g | Protein: 36 g | Fat: 2g

82

Red Pepper Cottage Cheese Dip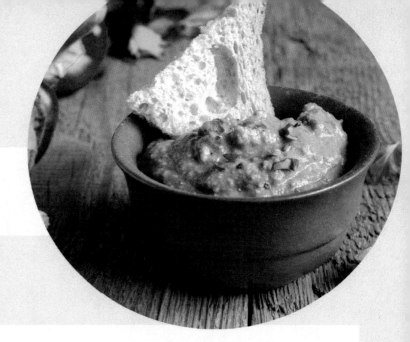

| SERVINGS:1 | PREPPING TIME: 5 MIN | COOKING TIME: 0 MIN |

INGREDIENTS

- 1/2 Cup Trader Joe's Red Pepper Spread
- 1/2 cup fat-free cottage cheese
- Fresh chopped parsley for garnish

DIRECTIONS

1. Mix red pepper dip with cottage cheese.
2. Immersion blend or add to a blender to whip until smooth
3. Sprinkle with fresh chopped parsley & enjoy with your favorite vegetables

Make this dip from Scratch by blending the following:

- 1 jar roasted red peppers
- 1 cup cherry tomatoes
- 2 garlic cloves (or 1.5 tsp minced garlic) roasted on a pan
- 1 T olive oil
- 1/2 tsp smoked paprika
- ½ tsp dried oregano
- 1 T salt, 1/2 tsp pepper

Calories per serving: 180 | Carbohydrate: 21g | Protein: 15g | Fat: 4g

TABLE OF CONTENTS

Turkey Bacon Wrapped Stuffed Dates

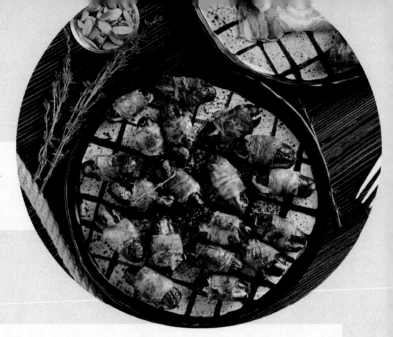

SERVINGS:1   PREPPING TIME: 10 MIN   COOKING TIME: 8 MIN

INGREDIENTS

- 3 pitted medjool dates
- 3 slices of turkey bacon (I love Boarshead)
- 1/4 cup part skim ricotta cheese

DIRECTIONS

1. Line a tray with parchament paper.
2. These are easier with pitted medjool dates but if you have to de-pit them, de-pit and spoon a tiny amount of ricotta in the center then gently encourage the two sides of the date closed. Ricotta will not be fully enclosed.
3. Wrap raw turkey bacon around the date and place the end of the turkey bacon side down onto parchment paper to hold it in place.
4. Airfry for 12-15 minutes at 375°F or bake for 15-20 minutes at 400F

Calories per serving (3 dates): 290 | Carbohydrate: 33g | Protein: 17g | Fat: 10g

Peach and "Burrata" Toast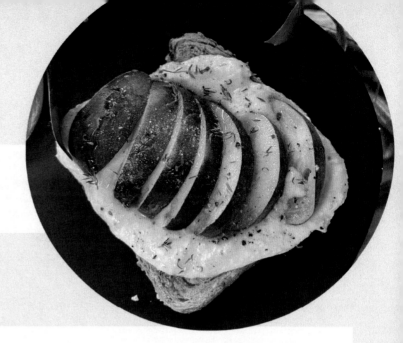

SERVINGS:1   PREPPING TIME: 10 MIN   COOKING TIME: 8 MIN

INGREDIENTS

- 1/2 ripe peach
- 1 slice of high-protein bread (I love Equii or Royo)
- 1/4 cup + 1/8 cup of low fat/fat-free cottage cheese, whipped
- 1/8 cup part skim ricotta cheese
- 1 tsp vanilla extract
- 2 thyme sprigs
- 1/2 tsp Hot Honey or regular honey

DIRECTIONS

1. Slice a peach in half and remove it's pits. Slice the peach into thin slices
2. In a small bowl mix ricotta, cottage cheese, and vanilla
3. Toast 2 pieces of bread (make sure it's really toasted so it doesn't get soggy!)
4. Spoon your cheese mixture on toasted bread then assemble peach slices on top
5. Drizzle honey over peaches and thyme leaves!

Calories: 260 | Carbohydrate: 35g | Protein: 24g | Fat: 3g

Everything But the Bagel Lox Rolls

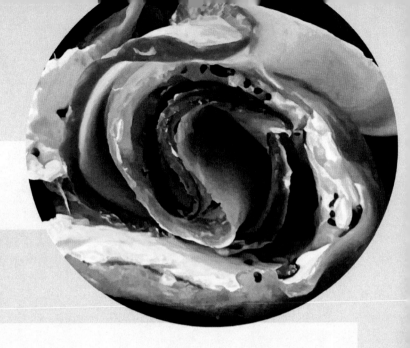

SERVINGS:4 ROLLS   PREPPING TIME: 10 MIN   COOKING TIME: 0 MIN

INGREDIENTS

- 8 oz smoked salmon (Everything but the Bagel seasoned is best!)
- 4 T lite cream cheese
- 4 thinly sliced peel of an english cucumber
- Everything but the Bagel Seasoning (for plain smoked salmon version)

DIRECTIONS

1. Cut an english cucumber in half.
2. Take a vegetable peeler and peel off the skin of the cucumber
3. With downward pressure, peel a very thin and flat layer of cucumber. Repeat 4 times for 4 thin, flat cucumber shavings.
4. Lay down 2 oz of smoked salmon on a clean surface
5. Smear with low fat cream cheese, season with Everything But the Bagel Seasoning (if needed) and layer the cucumber slice on top.
6. Begin to roll the entire strip of cucumber, salmon, and cream cheese into a small roll-up. Tuck the ends and place in a bowl. Repeat 3 more times!

Calories per roll: 118 | Carbohydrate: 2g | Protein: 15g | Fat: 6g

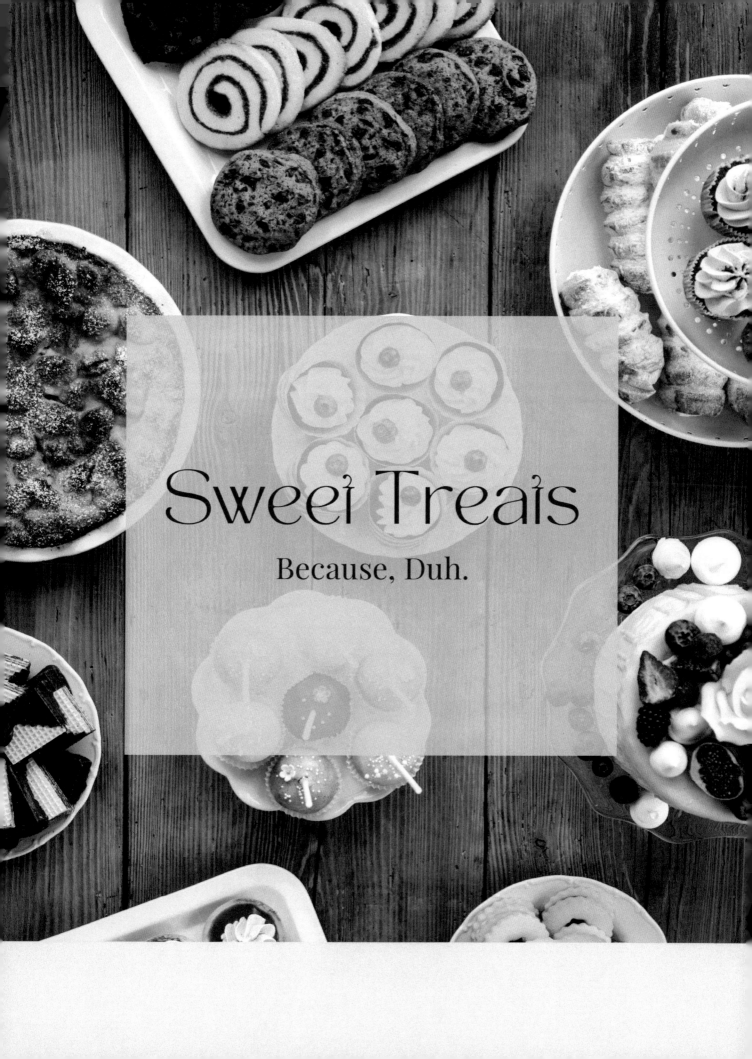

Sweet Treats

Because, Duh.

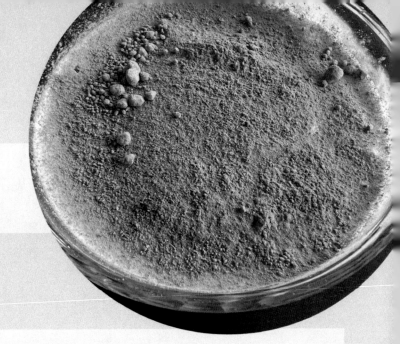

High-Protein Tiramisu

SERVINGS: 1-2   PREPPING TIME: 10 MIN   SETTING TIME: 20 MIN

INGREDIENTS

- 1 rice cake
- 1 Promix Nutrition Protein puff bar (or another rice cake, but will be less protein)
- 1 scoop vanilla protein powder I used Clean Simple Eats (code PROTEINSNACKQUEEN for 10% off
- 1/8 cup ricotta cheese, part skim
- 1/2 cup fat free greek yogurt
- 2 tsp sugar free sweetener (I used Lakanto!)
- 1 cup cold brew of choice
- Cocoa powder
- Coffee powder/grounds

DIRECTIONS

1. Pour coffee into a bowl. Dip a rice cake in it on both sides and place wet rice cake in another bowl.
2. In a separate bowl, mix yogurt, ricotta, protein powder, sweetener, a tsp coffee grounds.
3. Pour half if mixture over rice cake.
4. Layer promix bar on top then layer with the other half of the mixture.
5. Set in the fridge for 20 min to firm.
6. Sprinkle/dust with cocoa powder and coffee grounds and enjoy!

Calories for entire bowl: 424 | Carbohydrate: 43g | Protein: 49g | Fat: 6g

87

High-Protein Chocolate Strawberry Crepe

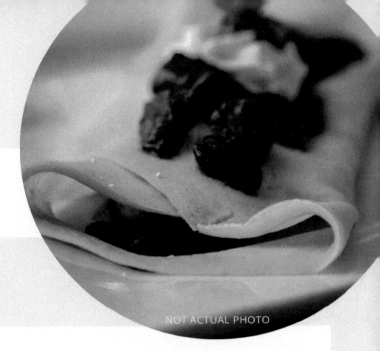

NOT ACTUAL PHOTO

SERVINGS: 1 CREPE   PREPPING TIME: 10 MIN   COOKING TIME: 0 MIN

INGREDIENTS

- 1 Egglife Cinnamon Wrap (You may use plain also)
- 1 scoop of Vanilla Protein Powder
- 5-10g sugar free, fat free chocolate pudding - I love Simply Delish
- 15g Cocoa powder
- 5 strawberries, chopped
- 1/2 cup almond milk
- 5g zero calorie sweetener (Swerve, Lakanto, Splenda)
- fat free whipped cream, I love Reddiwhip.
- Powdered sugar

DIRECTIONS

1. Chop your straberries!
2. Mix milk, protein powder, pudding powder, cocoa powder, & sweetener.
3. Lay the wrap flat and spoon chocolate filling into the middle.
4. Add 1/2 of the chopped strawberries on top.
5. Fold the wrap & sprinkle the rest of the strawberries on top.
6. Top with a spray of fat-free whipped cream and a sprinkle of powdered sugar!

Calories: 250 | Carbohydrate: 25g | Protein: 25g | Fat: 6g

High-Protein PB&J Tortilla

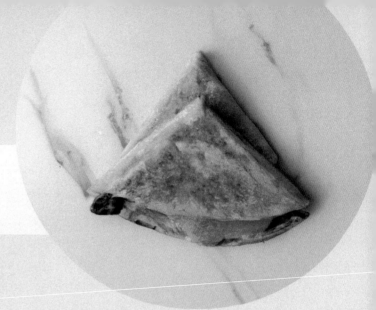

SERVINGS: 1
TORTILLA, 2 HALVES

PREPPING TIME: 10 MIN

COOKING TIME: 0 MIN

INGREDIENTS

- Your favorite high protein tortilla. I used <u>Hero.</u>
- 30g vanilla protein powder
- 2 T <u>PB2 Powder</u>
- 30g <u>Reduced Sugar Jam</u>
- 3 T water or almond milk

DIRECTIONS

1. Mix protein powder, PB2, and milk/water in a bowl to get a thick consistency.
2. Cut your tortilla in half.
3. Add protein mixture to one side
4. Smear jam on the other side.
5. Fold totrilla half in half & place both on a skillet to warm/toast.

Be mindful, heat can make mixture runny, and may cause mixture to ooze out.

Calories: 307 | Carbohydrate: 30g | Protein: 32g | Fat: 7g

High-Protein Birthday Cake Waffles

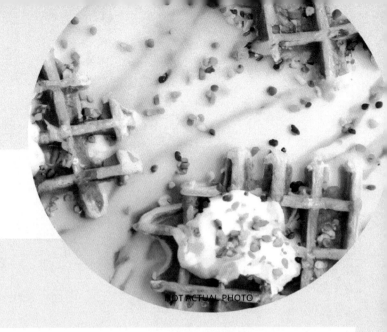

NOT ACTUAL PHOTO

SERVINGS: 1-2 WAFFLES DEPENDING ON WAFFLE MAKER SIZE!   PREPPING TIME: 5 MIN   COOKING TIME: 5 MIN

INGREDIENTS

- 1 scoop of birthday cake-flavored protein powder (I used Unico)
- 1/2 a mashed ripe banana
- 1 large egg
- 1 egg white or 2 T liquid egg whites
- 1/4 tsp baking powder
- 2 T plant milk to thin batter
- pinch of salt

Toppings:

- Sugar-free maple syrup (I use Lakanto!)
- Fat-free whipped cream
- Rainbow Sprinkles

DIRECTIONS

1. Whisk protein, banana, egg, eggwhites, salt, and baking powder in a bowl.
2. Add 1-2 T plant milk to thin batter if needed.
3. Grease a waffle maker with avocado oil
4. Pour half of the mixture in the center. BE VERY CAREFUL not to over-fill the waffle maker otherwise the batter will leak and create a mess!
5. Cook until waffle maker blinks green. Top with your favorite toppings!

Calories without toppings: 270 | Carbohydrate: 19g | Protein: 36g | Fat: 6g

Protein Strawberry Cheesecake

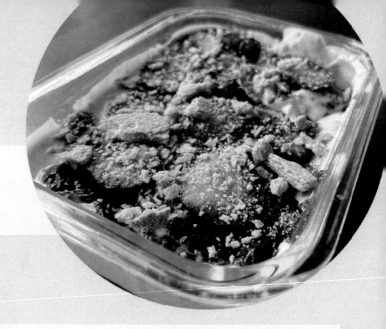

SERVINGS: 1-2   PREPPING TIME: 10 MIN   COOKING TIME: 0 MIN

INGREDIENTS

- 5 strawberries sliced
- 1 cup fat-free greek yogurt
- 1-2 T fat-free/low-fat cream cheese
- 15g Strawberry Pudding Mix (I used Simply Delish)
- Optional: 10g fat-free Cheesecake Pudding Mix
- 1 Scoop Vanilla protein powder
- 1/2 sheet crushed graham cracker
- 2 T Strawberry or Raspberry Preserves (I recommend GoodGood OR Reduced Sugar Raspberry Preserves from Trader Joe's!)
- Squeeze of half a lemon

DIRECTIONS

1. Lay sliced strawberries at the bottom of a medium sized bowl.
2. In a separate bowl, combine Greek yogurt, cream cheese, pudding mix, protein powder and lemon
3. Stir well!
4. Pour the mixture over the strawberries.
5. Warm fruit preserves in the microwave then spread it on top of cream mixture.
6. Add a few strawberry slices on top topped with crumbled graham crackers!

Calories for entire recipe: 350 | Carbohydrate: 46g | Protein: 40g | Fat: 4g

Apple Pie Mug Cake

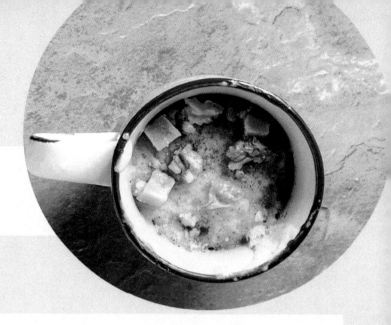

SERVINGS: 1   PREPPING TIME: 10 MIN   COOKING TIME: 1 MIN

INGREDIENTS

- 1/3 cup unsweetened apple sauce
- 1 scoop vanilla protein
- 1 T flour
- 1/4 of an apple, chopped small and cubed
- 1/2 tsp baking powder
- 1/2 tsp cinnamon powder
- Optional: Caramel Drizzle, Fat Free Whipped cream

DIRECTIONS

- Toss your apple pieces into a bowl with a dash of cinnamon and microwave for 1 minute to pre-cook.
- In a large mug, combine applesauce, protein powder, baking powder, flour, and cinnamon powder. Mix well - you may use a handheld milk frother!
- Add apple cubes and stir.
- Place in the microwave for about 60 seconds. The center should be somewhat gooey and soft.
- Add toppings as you'd like!

Calories without topping: 217 | Carbohydrate: 27g | Protein: 26g | Fat: 1g

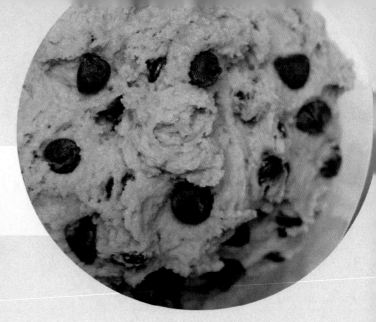

High-Protein Edible Cookie Dough

SERVINGS: 1   PREPPING TIME: 5 MIN   COOKING TIME: 0

INGREDIENTS

- 10 g vanilla pudding
- 5g chocolate pudding
- 70g fat-free cottage cheese
- 30g vanilla portein powder
- 1 T almond flour
- 1 T almond milk
- 1 T honey
- 1 T sugar-free chocolate chips (I love Enjoy Life!)

DIRECTIONS

- Add all ingredients except chocolate chips to a blender. Blend until smooth.
- Mix in chocolate chips and chill!
- Enjoy!

Calories without topping: 427 | Carbohydrate: 46g | Protein: 36g | Fat: 11g

Protein Fruit Bake Crumble

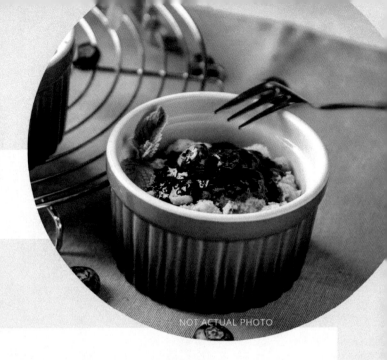

NOT ACTUAL PHOTO

SERVINGS: 1 BOWL   PREPPING TIME: 10 MIN   COOKING TIME: 5 MIN

INGREDIENTS

- 3/4 cup cinnamon protein cereal (Magic Spoon, Snack House, Three Wishes, Catalina Crunch)
- 1 scoop Vanilla Protein Powder
- 1/2 cup blueberries
- 1/4 cup chopped strawberries
- 2 T Lakanto Sugar Free Maple Syrup

DIRECTIONS

1. Grease a baking dish with oil.
2. Add cereal & protein powder.
3. Crush up mixture into a flour like consistency.
4. Add blueberries and top with 1 T sugar free syrup. Add a couple crumbs of cereal on top.
5. Airfry on 400F for 5 min
6. Add 1 T syrup on top after it's cooked.
7. Add a few chopped fresh strawberries.

Calories: 282 | Carbohydrate: 29g | Protein: 25g | Fat: 7g

Elvis Dumplings

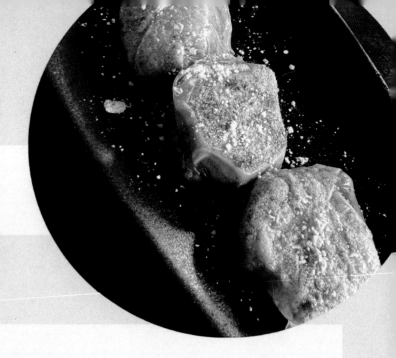

SERVINGS: 4 DUMBLINGS   PREPPING TIME: 10 MIN   COOKING TIME: 5 MIN

INGREDIENTS

- 2 rice paper sheets, sliced in half
- 20g Simply Delish Keto Chocolate Pudding Mix
- 1/2 banana sliced into 4 pieces
- 1 scoop chocolate protein powder (I used Quest)
- 2 T Pb2 powder
- 1/2 turkey bacon sliced into smal pieces

DIRECTIONS

1. Make the chocolate PB2 mixture by mixing pudding powder, PB2 powder, and protein powder with 2-3 T almond milk.
2. Dip a rice paper sheet into a plate of water for 1 second then remove and place on a flat surface. Slice in half.
3. Spoon a tablespoon of chocolate mixture onto the middle of a half. Then add banana and bacon.
4. Fold the ends of the wrap over and tuck under so there's no hole left for filling to get out.
5. Repeat 3 times.
6. Grease a skillet and turn to low heat.
7. Place dumplings on skillet, flipping on both sides until each side gets crispy.
8. Dust with powdered sugar and enjoy!

Calories per dumpling: 90 | Carbohydrate: 12g | Protein: 8g | Fat: 0g

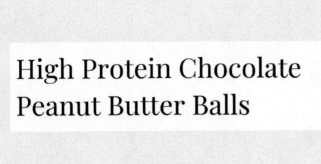
High Protein Chocolate Peanut Butter Balls

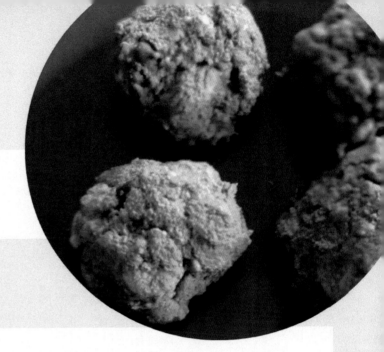

SERVINGS: 6 BALLS   PREPPING TIME: 7 MIN   COOK TIME: 0 MIN

INGREDIENTS

- 1 brown rice cake
- 2 T PB2 powder
- 30g protein powder of choice (vanilla, chocolate or Peanut butter will all be good!)
- 1 T chocolate chips (I use Enjoy Life)
- 3-4T water or plant milk
- Pinch of salt
- (You can add any Maple Syrup or zero calorie sweetener if you'd like it to be more sweet!)

DIRECTIONS

1. Mix all dry ingredients together then slowly add cold water or plant milk until consistency becomes like a batter. The more liquid you add, the stickier the balls will be.
2. Roll into 6 balls and place in the fridge for at least 30 minutes to harden.

Calories for 6 balls: 324 | Carbohydrate: 33g | Protein: 30g | Fat: 8g

Protein S'Mores Bowl

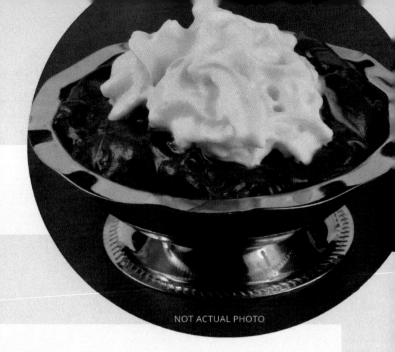

NOT ACTUAL PHOTO

SERVINGS: 1   PREPPING TIME: 5 MIN   COOKING TIME: 0 MIN

INGREDIENTS

- 1.5 sheets of graham crackers
- 1 scoop of vanilla protein powder
- 1/4 box of Simply Delish Chocolate keto pudding powder
- 4 T Toasted Marshmallow Coconut Creamer (you can sub some marshmallows here and just use almond milk if this is hard to find
- Fat free reddiwhip

DIRECTIONS

1. Crumble/pulverize 1 sheet of graham crackers
2. In a separate bowl, mix pudding, protein, and milk/creamer
3. Fill the bottom of a small bowl with graham cracker crumbles
4. Spoon filling on top and smoothen mixture to be level
5. Crumble half a sheet of graham cracker
6. Spray whipped cream on top
7. Sprinkle 1/2 sheet crumbled graham cracker on top and ENJOY!

Calories: 315 | Carbohydrate: 36g | Protein: 27g | Fat: 7g

97

Vanilla Ricotta Blintz

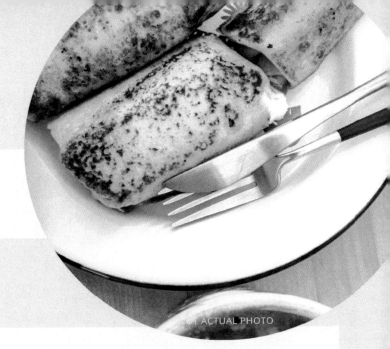

ACTUAL PHOTO

SERVINGS: 1   PREPPING TIME: 5-10 MIN   COOKING TIME: 6 MIN

INGREDIENTS

- 1/4 cup part skim ricotta cheese
- 1/2 scoop vanilla protein powder
- 1 Twin Dragon Egg roll wrapper
- 2 tsp Lakanto Monk Fruit Golden (or any other low calorie sweetener)
- 1/2 tsp vanilla extract

DIRECTIONS

1. Blend ricotta, protein, and 1 tsp Lakanto golden powder with vanilla extract.
2. Lay an eggroll wrapper on a flat surface with a bowl of water nearby.
3. Spoon mixture into center of wrapper.
4. Wet the edges of the egg roll wrapper so they stick when wrapping.
5. Fold the sides to completely enclose the filling and fold the edges over.
6. Airfry at 380°F for 6 min.
7. Spray a little oil on top and sprinkle Monk Fruit Golden on top, or dip in a bowl of Monk Fruit Golden!
8. ENJOY!

Calories: 260 | Carbohydrate: 29g | Protein: 27g | Fat: 4g

Banana Cream Pie Bowl

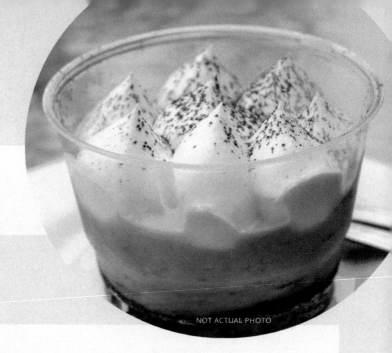

NOT ACTUAL PHOTO

SERVINGS: 1   **PREPPING TIME: 5 MIN**   **COOKING TIME: 0 MIN**

INGREDIENTS

- 1.5 sheets of graham crackers
- 1/2 T melted butter
- 1 scoop of vanilla protein powder
- 1/4 box of <u>Simply Delish Banana Keto Pudding</u> powder
- 4 T milk of choice
- Fat-free whipped cream, I'm using Reddi whip
- 1/4 banana, sliced in small discs

DIRECTIONS

1. Crumble/pulverize 1 sheet of graham crackers (you canplace it in a snack bag and use a rolling pin or water bottle)
2. Melt 5 g of butter in the microwave. In a separate bowl, mix pudding, protein, and milk
3. Fill the bottom of a small bowl with graham cracker crumbles & butter and stir! Pat down so you have a firm crust.
4. In a separate bowl, mix pudding, protein, and milk/creamer.
5. Spoon filling on top and smoothen mixture to be level
6. Crumble half a sheet of graham cracker
7. Spray whipped cream on top!
8. Top with 1/2 sheet crumbled graham cracker & banana slices.

Calories: 360 | Carbohydrate: 43g | Protein: 27g | Fat: 9g

High-Protein Monkey Bread

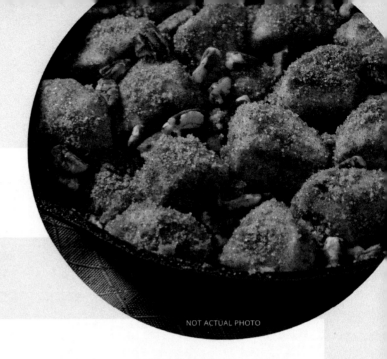

NOT ACTUAL PHOTO

SERVINGS: 7 BALLS   PREPPING TIME: 10 MIN   COOKING TIME: 8-15 MIN

INGREDIENTS

- 1 cup all purpose flour
- 1/2 cup vanilla or cinnamon protein powder (casein works BEST)
- 3/4 cup fat-free Greek yogurt
- 2 T 0 calorie sweetener(swerve)
- 1 T almond milk
- 1/2 T baking powder
- 1/2 T cinnamon
- 1 T butter
- 1 T powdered cane sugar
- 1 T 0 calorie sweetener of choice (I used swerve)
- Optional glaze: 1/4 C (36g) powdered sugar (I used Swerve Confectioners*) with 3-4 tsp water and pour over the top.

DIRECTIONS

1. Combine flour, protein, yogurt, sweetener, almond milk, and cinnamon in a bowl and stir . Be sure not to over-stir! You should get a dough-like consistency!
2. In a separate bowl, combine melted butter, powdered sugar, cinnamon, & 0 calorie sweetener
3. On a flat open surface, sprinkle some flour & separate the dough, rolling each piece into balls
4. Dip and roll each ball in butter and sugar mixture and place closely together in an airfryer tray to create 7 balls stuck together You may also use an oven.
5. Airfry at 350F for 8-10 min or bake in the oven at 350F for 10-15 min.

Calories per ball with coating & without sugar glaze:
125 | Carbohydrate: 18g | Protein: 10g | Fat: 2g

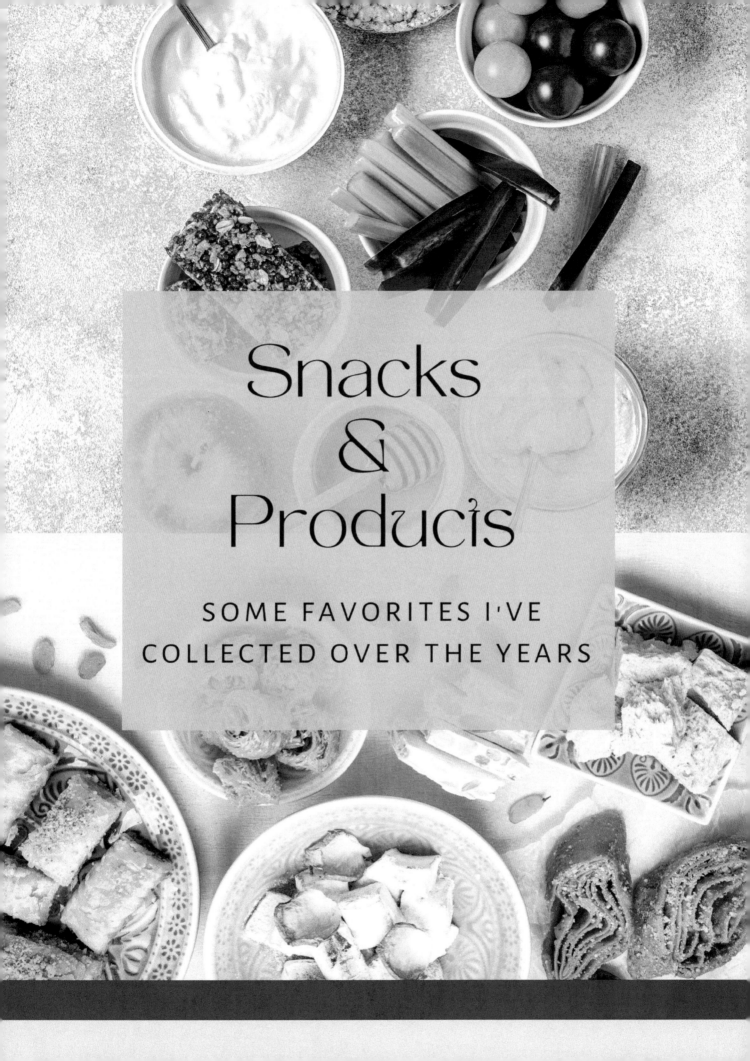

Snacks & Products

SOME FAVORITES I'VE COLLECTED OVER THE YEARS

BREAKFAST PRODUCTS

Sweets

- <u>BIRCHBENDERS PROTEIN PANCAKE & WAFFLE MIX</u> - [1.75OZ - 180 CAL: 1.5F, 26C, 16P] *FOUND AT WF*
- <u>BIRCHBENDERS PALEO BANANA PANCAKE AND WAFFLE MIX</u> [1.25OZ - 140 CAL - 6F, 18C, 6P]
- <u>LEGENDARY FOODS TASTY PASTRY</u> - [180 CAL: 7F, 24C, 20P]
- <u>PAMCAKES PANCAKE MIX</u> [1.25OZ - 130 CAL: 4.5F, 10C, 12P]
- <u>VIKING WAFFLES</u> - 20G PROTEIN PER WAFFLE!

Syrups & Jams

- <u>LAKANTO SUGAR FREE MONKFRUIT MAPLE SYRUP</u>
- <u>AGAVE 5 LOW GLYCEMIC SWEETENER</u>
- <u>GOOD GOOD NO SUGAR ADDED JAM</u>
- <u>LAKANTO GOLDEN MONK FRUIT SWEETENER</u>

Savory

- <u>GOOD FOOD MADE SIMPLE BREAD-LESS TURKEY & EGG SANDWICH</u>
- <u>GOOD FOOD MADE SIMPLE EGG WHITE PATTIES</u>
- <u>BILINSKI'S SPICY ITALIAN CHICKEN SAUSAGE</u> - 1 SAUSAGE - 90 CAL: 3F, 1C, 14P
- <u>AMLYU CHICKEN SAUSAGE</u> - [1 SAUSAGE - 100 CAL: 5F, 1C, 12P]
- <u>APPLEGATE ORGANIC TURKEY BACON</u> - 1 SLICE - 30 CAL: 0F, 0C, 5
- <u>BOARSHEAD TURKEY BACON</u>
- <u>AMLYU CHICKEN BURGERS</u> - 1 PATTY: 170 CAL: 8F, 2C, 22P
- <u>EGGWICH BREAKFAST SANDWICH</u> - 1 SANDWICH: 190 CAL, 17G P

BREAKFAST PRODUCTS

Cereals

- <u>SNACK HOUSE KETO CEREAL, ANY FLAVOR</u>- CODE PROTEINSNACKQUEEN SAVES YOU $ [1 CUP - 115 CAL: 5F, 8C, 15P]
- <u>THREE WISHES PROTEIN CEREAL,</u> - [1 CUP - 120 CAL: 2F, 18C, 8P] VEGAN, GF*
- <u>CATALINA CRUNCH PROTEIN CEREAL,</u> - [1 CUP - 110 CAL: 6F, 14C, 11P] FOUND AT WF |VEGAN, GF*
- <u>MAGIC SPOON PROTEIN CEREAL,</u> - [1 CUP - 140 CAL: 7F, 15C, 13P] GF
- <u>KODIAK CAKES HIGH PROTEIN OATMEAL</u> - [1 PACKET: 180 CAL: 2.5F, 31C, 12P]

Yogurts

- <u>STONEYFIELD ORGANIC GRASS FED FAT FREE GREEK YOGURT</u> - [¾ CUP - 90 CAL: 0F, 7C, 16P] FOUND AT WHOLE FOODS & TARGET
- <u>CHOBANI 0% FAT GREEK YOGURT</u> - [¾ CUP - 90 CAL: 0F, 6C, 16P]
- <u>SIGGI'S 0% MILK FAT NORDIC YOGURT</u> - [¾ CUP - 100 CAL: 0F, 6C, 17P] FOUND AT WHOLE FOODS
- <u>SIGGI'S PLANT-BASED COCONUT BLEND YOGURT</u> [180 CAL: 11F, 11C, 10P] VEGAN
- <u>KITEHILL PLANT-BASED GREEK STYLE YOGURT</u> - [140 CAL: 6F, 4C 17P]
- <u>MAPLE HILL WHOLE FAT GRASSFED YOGURT</u> - [¾ CUP - 150 CAL: 7F, 9C, 15P]
- <u>GOOD CULTURE COTTAGE CHEESE</u> - [150 G - 140 CAL: 4F, 6C, 19P]

Pasta

VERY LOW CAL

- <u>WONDER NOODLES</u> [o CALORIES] *VEGAN, GF*
- <u>MIRACLE NOODLES</u> [3 OZ - 5 CAL: oF, 3C, oP] *VEGAN, GF*
- <u>KELP NOODLES</u> [4 OZ - 6 CAL: oF, 3C, oP] *VEGAN, GF*
- TRADER JOE'S HEARTS OF PALM PASTA NOODLES [3 OZ - 20 CAL: oF, 4 C,1P] *VEGAN, GF*
- <u>PALMINI HEARTS OF PALM LINGUINE</u> [3 OZ - 20 CAL: oF, 4 C,1P] *VEGAN, GF*
- <u>PALMINI HEARTS OF PALM LASAGNA</u> [3 OZ - 20 CAL: oF, 4 C,1P *VEGAN, GF*

LOW CAL:

- <u>CARB-NADA REDUCED CARB PASTA NOODLES</u> [2 OZ - 170 CAL: 1.5F, 27C, 15P] *VEGETARIAN*
- <u>EXPLORE ASIAN BLACK BEAN & EDAMAME PASTA</u> [2OZ - 180 CAL: 3.5F, 20C, 24P] *VEGAN, GF*
- *<u>KAIZEN HIGH PROTEIN PLANT BASED PASTA</u>*
- <u>PASTABILITIES</u>

HEALTHIER THAN THE TRADITIONAL:

- <u>BANZA CHICKPEA PASTA</u> [2OZ - 190 CAL: 3F, 35C, 11P]
- TRADER JOE'S TRUFFLE MUSHROOM RAVIOLI [1 CUP - 190 CAL: 8F, 20C, 8P]
- TRADER JOE'S CAULIFLOWER GNOCCHI [1 CUP - 140 CAL: 3F, 22C, 2P]

TIP #1: MIX LOW CARB NOODLES WITH REGULAR NOODLES IF YOU'RE LOOKING FOR SOMETHING MORE SUBSTANTIAL BUT WITHOUT THE ADDED CALORIES.

Pasta Sauce

- <u>CUCINA ANTICA NONNA'S RECIPE PASTA SAUCE</u> [½ CUP - 50 CAL: 1.5F, 9C, 1P]
- <u>YO MAMA KETO MARINARA PASTA SAUCE</u> [½ CUP - 60 CAL: 4.5F, 5C, 1P]

TIP #2: TO ADD MORE PROTEIN & FLAVOR, ADD LEAN GROUND BEEF TO THE SAUCE. CONSIDER BAKING CHICKEN BREAST AS AN ALTERNATIVE, AND LOWER FAT OPTION.

TIP #3: TO ADD VEGETABLES, ADD VEGGIES OF CHOICE! FRESH HERBS ARE ALWAYS A PLUS.

Lunch & Dinner Products

Rice

VERY LOW CAL:

- <u>WONDER NOODLES RICE</u> [0 CALORIES] VEGAN, GF*
- <u>MIRACLE RICE</u> [3 OZ - 10 CAL: 0F, 3C, 0P] VEGAN, GF*

LOW CARB:

- CAULIFLOWER RICE - FROZEN OR REFRIGERATED IN MOST GROCERY STORES. VEGAN, GF*
- TRADER JOE'S FROZEN CAULIFLOWER FRIED RICE [1 CUP - 50 CAL: 2F, 7C, 2P] VEGAN, GF*
- TRADER JOE'S FROZEN SPICY MEXICAN STYLE CAULIFLOWER RICE [1 CUP - 50 CAL: 2.5F, 5C, 2P] VEGAN*
- <u>RITE RICE</u> [1.5OZ - 180 CAL: 2F, 30C, 10P] FOUND AT WF, VEGAN, GF*
- <u>ORGANIC RICED CAULIFLOWER STIRFRY</u> BY TATTOOED CHEF, AT TARGET

HEALTHIER THAN THE TRADITIONAL:

- TRADER JOE'S FROZEN ASPARAGUS RISOTTO [1 CUP - 160 CAL: 4F, 26C, 4P]
- <u>BANZA CHICKPEA RICE</u> [2 OZ - 180 CAL: 3F, 30C, 12P] VEGAN, GF*

Frozen Meals

- <u>CAULI'FLOUR FOODS CHICKEN ENCHILADA BAKE</u> - [1 ENTREE: 290 CAL: 16F, 17C, 21P] GF*
- <u>CAULI'FLOUR FOODS VEGGIE LASAGNA</u> - [1 ENTREE: 330 CAL: 21F, 15C, 24P] GF*
- <u>AMYLU CHICKEN BURGERS</u> - [1 PATTY: 170 CAL: 8F, 2C, 22P]
- <u>TRADER JOE'S CHICKEN ASADA DISH</u>
- <u>TRADER JOE'S CHICKEN SHU MAI</u>
- <u>TRADER JOE'S VEGAN BOLOGNESE</u>
- <u>KEVIN'S MEALS</u>

Breads & Tortillas

SANDWICH / BURGER BREADS:

- OUTER AISLE CAULIFLOWER SANDWICH THINS - [1 THIN - 50 CAL: 2.5F, 4C, 2P] FOUND AT WF. GF*
- EQUII SUPERSEED HIGH PROTEIN BREAD
- CARBONAUGHT BREAD - [1 SLICE - 80 CAL: 3.5F, 8C, 6P]
- CARBONAUGHT HAMBURGER BUNS - [1 BUN - 160 CAL: 6F, 15C, 11P]
- TRADER JOE'S CAULIFLOWER THINS - [1 THIN - 50 CAL: 2.5F, 1.5C, 4.5P] GF*
- ROYO LOW CARB, HIGH FIBER BREAD - [1 SLICE - 30 CAL,, 11G FIBER] CODE: PROTEINSNACKQUEEN
- ROYO LOW CARB EVERYTHING BAGEL - [1 BAGEL- 80 CAL] CODE: PROTEINSNACKQUEEN
- GLUTEN FREE PAGEL 250 CALORIES - 4G PROTEIN, 43G CARBS, 8G FAT
- THE BETTER BAGEL - 160 CALORIES, 26G PROTEIN, 40G CARBS, 2G FAT
- ZERO CARB BAGEL 90 CALORIES, 14G PROTEIN, 14G CARBS, 4 G FAT

TORTILLAS:

- TRADER JOE'S CARB SAVVY MINI TORTILLAS - [1 TORTILLA - 45 CALORIES: 1.5F, 9C, 4P]
- LA FACTORY LOW CARB TORTILLAS - [1 TORTILLA - 50 CAL: 2F, 11C, 5P]
- MISSION CARB BALANCE FLOUR TORTILLAS - [1 TORTILLA - 70 CAL: 3F, 19C, 5P]
- CAULIPOWER GRAIN FREE TORTILLAS - 1 TORTILLA - 70 CAL: 2F, 10C, 3.5P] GF*
- MISSION HIGH PROTEIN TORTILLA - 1 TORTILLA - 70 CAL: 3F, 15C, 7P]
- HERO TORTILLAS
- EGGLIFE EGG TORTILLAS & EGGLIFE CINNAMON TORTILLA
- LA TORTILLA FACTORY HIGH PROTEIN TORTILLA - 1 TORTILLA - 70 CAL: 2F, 10C, 3.5P

Lunch & Dinner Products

Pizza Crusts/ Pizzas:

- ~~KRUST CAULIFLOWER PIZZA CRUSTS - [⅓ CRUST - 40 CAL: 3F, 1C, 3P]~~
- TRADER JOE'S CAULIFLOWER PIZZA CRUSTS - [1 CRUST - 120 CAL: 6F, 4C, 10P]
- CAULIPOWER PIZZA - [½ PIZZA - 370 CAL: 15F, 44C, 13P] FOUND AT WF | GLUTEN FREE*
- QUEST THIN CRUST PIZZA - [⅓ PIZZA - 260 CAL: 17F, 18C, 20P]
- DAIYA DAIRY FREE, GLUTEN FREE CAULIFLOWER PIZZA - [¼ PIZZA - 300 CAL: 11F, 46C, 4P] FOUND AT WF | VEGAN*

Dressings & Dips

- SALSA VERDE, ITALIAN)
- SKINNY GIRL ITALIAN DRESSING
- NOBLE MADE CLASSIC BBQ - [2 T- 35 CAL - 0F, 8C, 0P]
- NOBLE MADE MUSTARD BBQ - [2T - 15 CAL - 0F, 3C, 0P]
- CALORIE FREE DRESSINGS BY WALDEN FARMS + RANCH & HONEY DIJON
- HELLMAN'S LOW FAT MAYO
- TRADER JOE'S SPINACH AND KALE GREEK YOGURT DIP - [1 OZ - 30 CAL: 2F, 2C, 1P]
- TRADER JOE'S VEGAN TZATZIKI DIP [1 OZ - 50 CAL: 4.5F, 2C, 0P]
- TRADER JOE'S GARLIC AND EGGPLANT DIP - [1 OZ - 30 CAL: 2F, 4C, 0P] - VEGAN*
- TRADER JOE'S EVERYTHING BUT THE ELOTE DIP [1 OZ - 60 CAL: 4F, 4C, 1P]

SNACKS

- QUEST NUTRITION PROTEIN CHIPS [ALL FLAVORS] - [1 BAG - 140 CAL: 4.5F, 4C, 20P]
- QUEST BARS
- QUEST CHIPS CHEESE CRACKERS
- PRIME BITES PROTEIN BROWNIES [1 BROWNIE - 190 CA: 7F, 25C, 16P]
- EAT ME GUILT FREE BROWNIES - [1 BROWNIE - 180 CA: 6F, 7C, 22P]
- PEA PROTEIN CRISPS- VEGAN
- CATALINA CRUNCH SNACK MIX [120CAL PER OZ: 7F, 9C,8P]
- LESSER EVIL SNACKS HIMALAYAN PINK SALT POPCORN [ALL FLAVORS] - [3 CUPS - 116 CAL: 4F, 17C, 4F] *FOUND AT WF | VEGAN**
- BEANFIELDS CHIPS - [1 OZ - 130 CAL: 6F, 16C, 4P] - | *VEGAN & GF**
- QUEVOS EGG WHITE CRISPS (LOCAL TO CHICAGO) - [1 OZ - 140 CAL: 10F**, 8C, 8P] | GF
- ASHAPOPS - [1 OZ - 100 CAL: 2F, 17C, 4P]
- FULFIL VITAMIN & PROTEIN BARS - [1 BAR - 160 CAL: 5F, 15C, 15P] DAIRYFREE*
- BARBELLS PROTEIN BARS - [1 BAR - 200 CAL: 7F, 20C, 20P]
- BLUEBERRY DARK CHOCOLATE PROTEIN BAR -[1 BAR - 230 CAL - 8F, 23C, 15P]
- HA! CHURRO FLAVORED CRUNCHERS - [1 PACK - 140 CAL -3.5F 17C, 11P]
- IWON CARAMELIZED ONION PUFFS

JERKY

- CHOMPS MEAT STICKS
- LORISSA'S KITCHEN BEEF STICKS, BEEF & CHICKEN JERKY - USE CODE SNACKQUEEN25 FOR 25% OFF YOUR ORDER
- COUNTRY ARCHER JERKY

Desserts & Candy

Links

- EAT ME GUILT FREE BROWNIES - [1 BROWNIE - 180 CA: 6F, 7C, 22P] GF

- PRIME BITES PROTEIN BROWNIES (I LIKE THEM BETTER THAN EAT ME GUILT FREE!) [1 BROWNIE - 190 CAL: 6F, 24C, 17P]

- LEGENDARY FOODS TASTY PASTRY - [180 CAL: 7F, 24C, 20P]

- SMART CAKES - [38 CALORIES PER CAKE]

- SMART MUFF'N [113 CALORIES PER MUFFIN: 8P, 9F, 20C]

- OATMEAL PROTEIN PIE - [320 CAL: 16F, 35C, 15P]

- CATALINA CRUNCH SANDWICH COOKIES - [90 CALORIES PER 2 COOKIES: 6F, 11C, 4P] **OREO LOVER

- LEGENDARYFOODS PROTEIN CINNAMON BUN - [200 CALORIES: 10F, 22C, 20P] *GF

- SINLESS MARSHMALLOW CRISP - [80 CALORIES: 3.5F, 13C, 8P] *GF

- PROMIX PROTEIN CRISP BARS

- TIDBITS LOW CALORIE MERINGUES

- SIMPLY DELISH SUGAR FREE KETO PUDDING MIX

- HEALTHY DESSERT IDEA: CRUMBLED UP EAT ME GUILT FREE BROWNIE (I LOVE THE BIRTHDAY CAKE FLAVOR), FROZEN BERRIES, AND FAT FREE REDDI WHIP WHIPPED CREAM!

- SHAMELESS GUMMIES - MULTIFLAVOR - 70 CALORIES PER BAG!

- SMART SWEETS LOW SUGAR, LOW CALORIE, HIGH FIBER GUMMY CANDY - MY FAVE - HIGH FIBER***

- CHOCO-RITE SUGAR FREE CHOCOLATE CARAMELS - [1 PACKAGE OF 2: 70 CALORIES: 4F, 14C] HIGH FIBER***

- BEHAVE HIGH FIBER LOW SUGAR GUMMY CANDY - 60 CALORIES PER BAG: 0F, 32C, 4P & 13 FIBER]

- PROJECT 7 LOW CALORIE FIBER SOUR GUMMY WORMS - 60 CAL PER BAG [37C, 18 G FIBER]

Icecream

- <u>HALO TOP ICE CREAM</u> - [1 PINT = 280-360 CALORIES. ½ CUP - 80 CAL: 2.5F, 16C, 5P] FOUND AT WF
- <u>ARCTIC ZERO ICE CREAM PINTS</u> [VEGAN] [1 PINT = 160 CALORIES: 0F, 28C, 12P] - AMAZON FRESH
- <u>FRONEN - ONLY 5 INGREDIENTS, DAIRY FREE ICE CREAM</u> - [½ CUP - 90 CAL: 4.5F, 15C, 2P] FOUND AT WF | V, GF*
- <u>ENLIGHTENED LIGHT ICE CREAM PINTS</u> - 280 - 400 CALORIES PER PINT
- <u>ENLIGHTENED FUDGE BARS</u> - [1 BAR - 70 CALORIES]
- <u>ENLIGHTENED DAIRY FREE**** ICE CREAM PINTS AND BARS</u> - 280 - 400 CALORIES PER PINT, 70 CALORIES PER BAR
- <u>ENLIGHTENED CHEESECAKE</u> - 180-220 CALORIES PER SMALL CAKE
- <u>ENLIGHTENED DOUGH BITES</u> - 200-300 CALORIES PER BAG
- <u>SUGAR FREE AND FAT FREE PUDDING</u> - CHOCOLATE & BANANA CREAM PIE FLAVORS ARE MY FAVORITE
- <u>YASSO CHOCOLATE COVERED VANILLA YOGURT POPPABLES</u> - 60 CALORIES PER POPPABLE, 350 CALORIES FOR THE WHOLE BOX (6 POPPABLES)
- <u>YASSO VANILLA BEAN ICECREAM SANDWICHES</u> - 100 CALORIES [4P, 20C, 1.5F]

Drinks

- ZEVIA COLA - SUGAR FREE, CALORIE FREE, STEVIA SWEETENED
- SPARKLING ICE ANTIOXIDANTS & VITAMINS SPARKLING WATER - SUGAR FREE, 5 CALORIES
- OLLIPOP PREBIOTIC SOFT DRINK - [BEST FLAVORS 1. STRAWBERRY VANILLA 2. CHERRY VANILLA 3. ORANGE CRUSH]
- QUEST PROTEIN SHAKE (DELICIOUS COFFEE CREAMER)
- KOIA PROTEIN SHAKES - TONS OF FLAVORS & FOUND AT WHOLE FOODS- VEGAN & GLUTEN FREE
- POPPI PREBIOTIC SODA
- SLATE HIGH PROTEIN CHOCOLATE MILK & COFFEE VARIETY
- FAIRLIFE HIGH PROTEIN DRINK

Protein Powders

- GAINFUL PERFORMANCE PROTEIN POWDER
- CLEAN SIMPLE EATS - PROTEINSNACKQUEEN FOR 10% OFF
- UNICO NUTRITION (I GET THE BIRTHDAY CUPCAKE FLAVOR)
- NAKED WHEY - VANILLA FLAVOR - CLEAN FLAVOR AND GOES WITH EVERYTHING
- OUTWORK NUTRITION BUILD PROTEIN IN CHOCOLATE OR VANILLA - THE CHOCOLATE FLAVOR IS DELICIOUS
- QUEST CHOCOLATE MILKSHAKE PROTEIN POWDER
- QUEST MULTI PURPOSE PROTEIN POWDER
- CORE PREFORM PLANT PROTEIN